I0711001

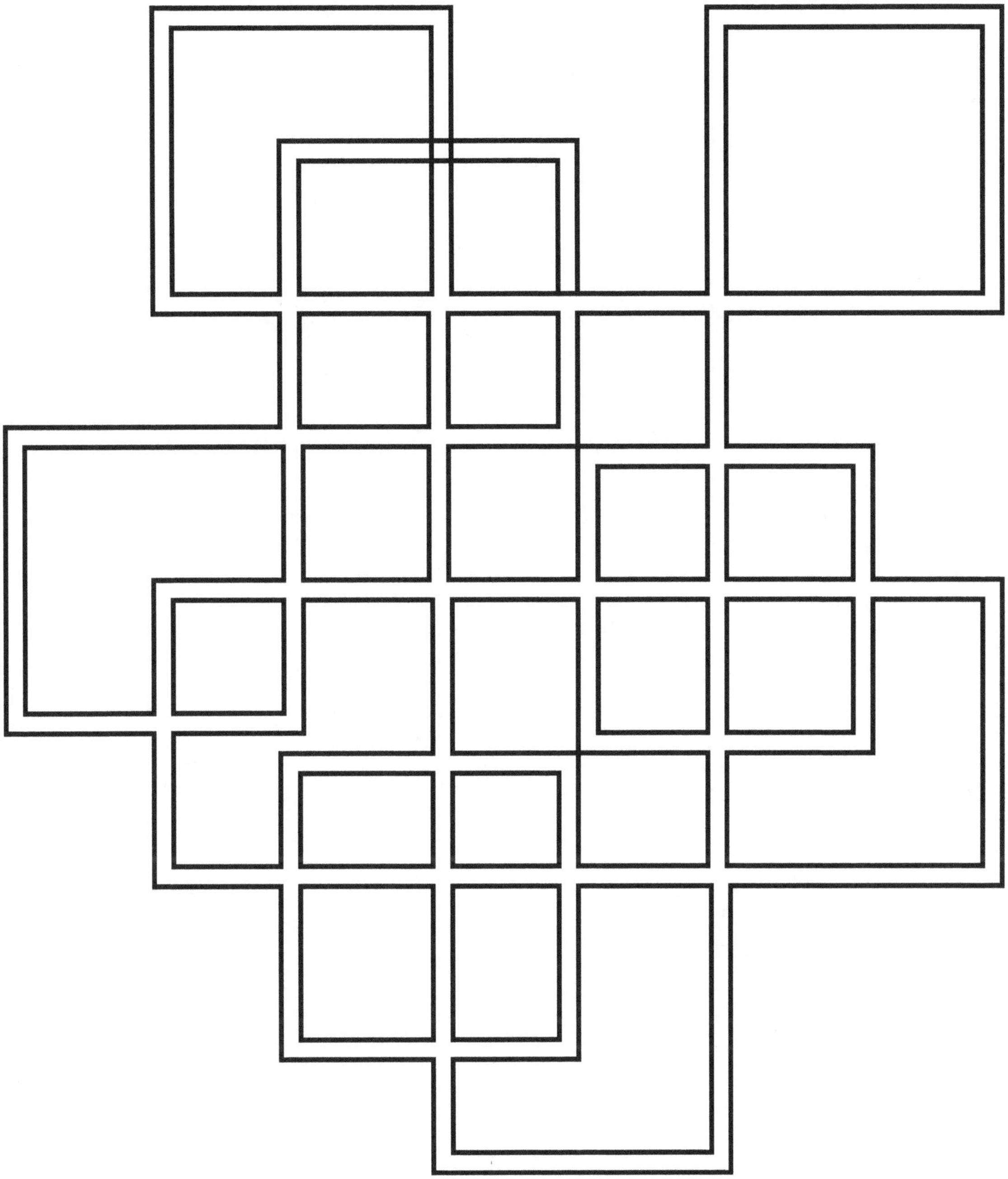

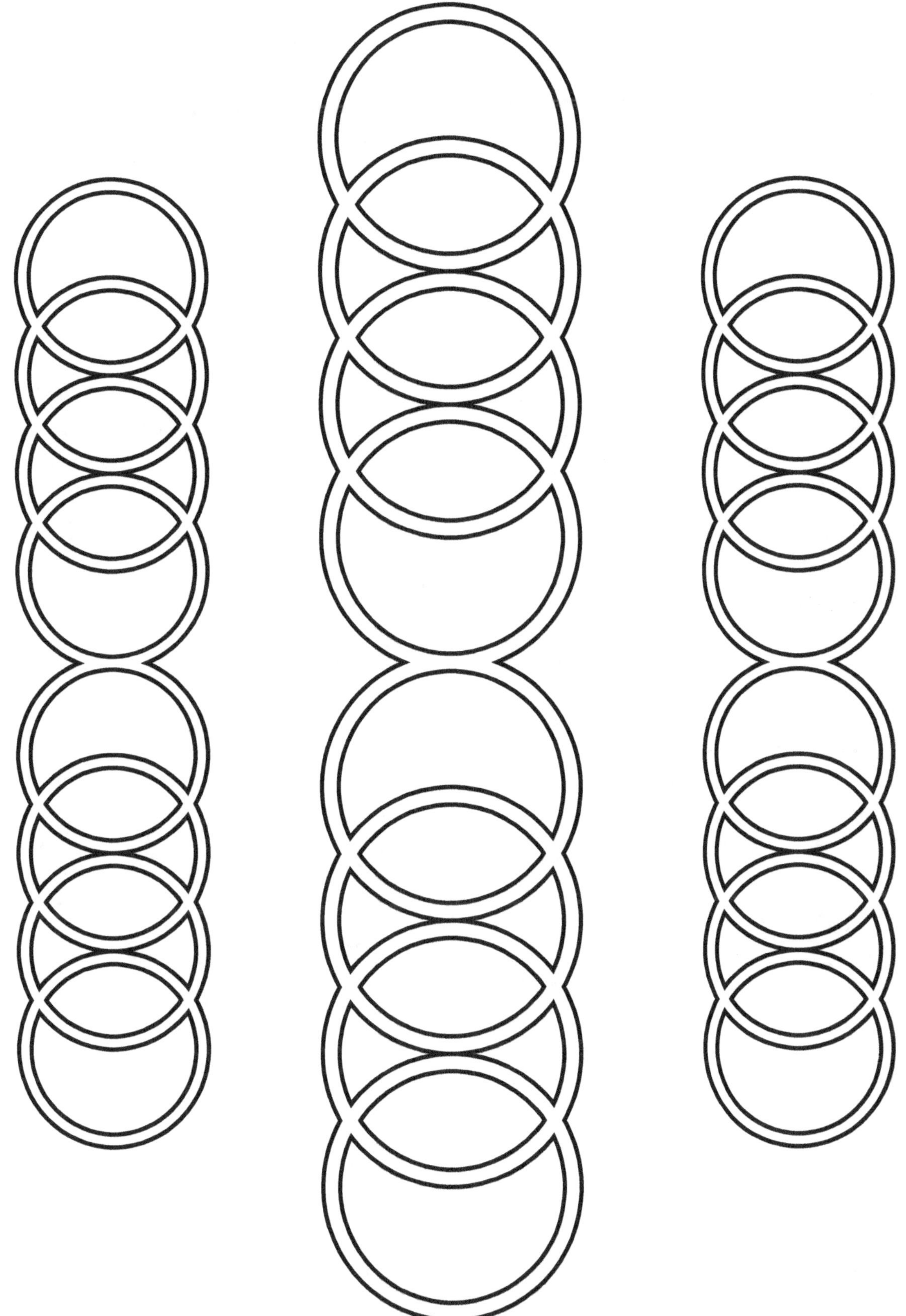

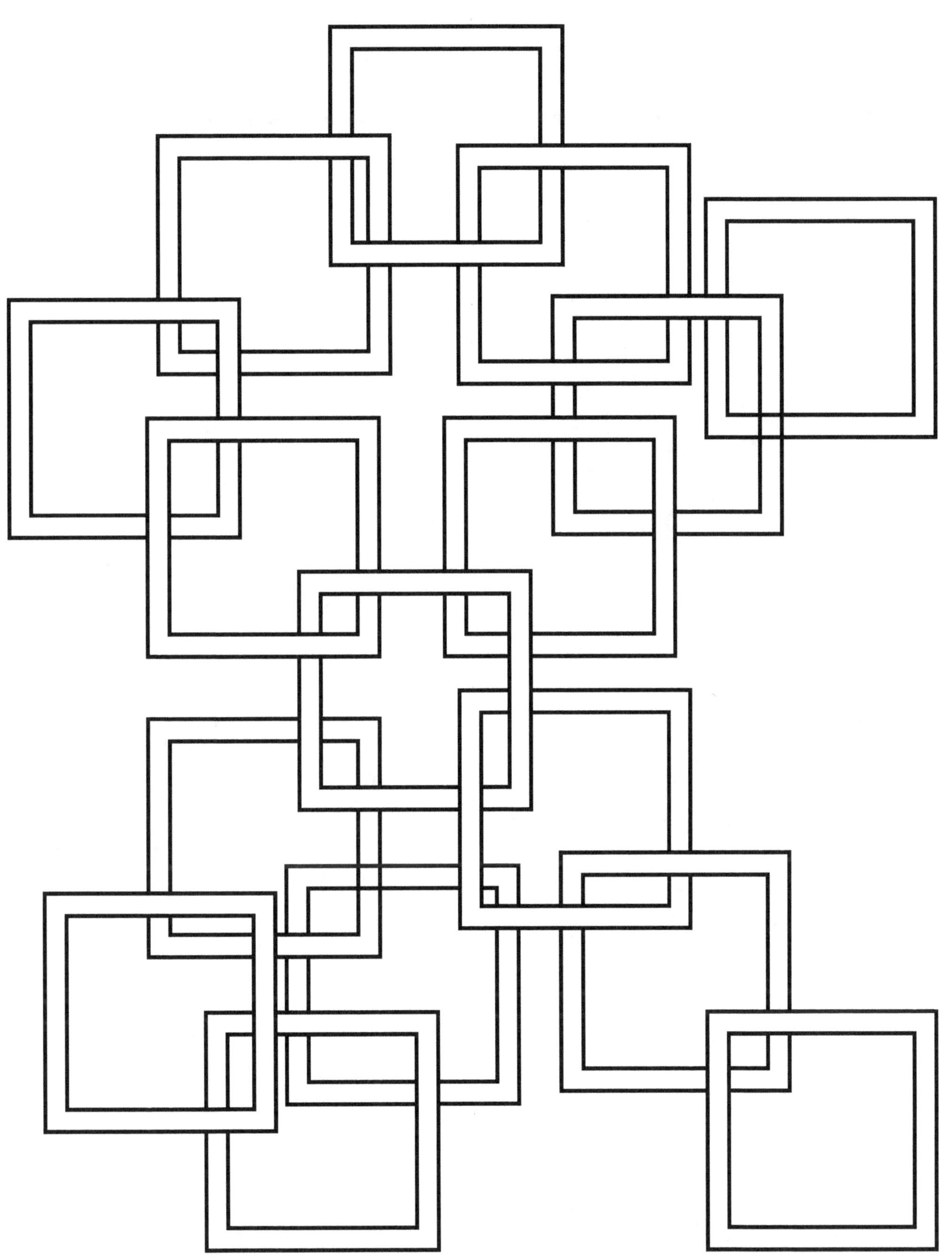

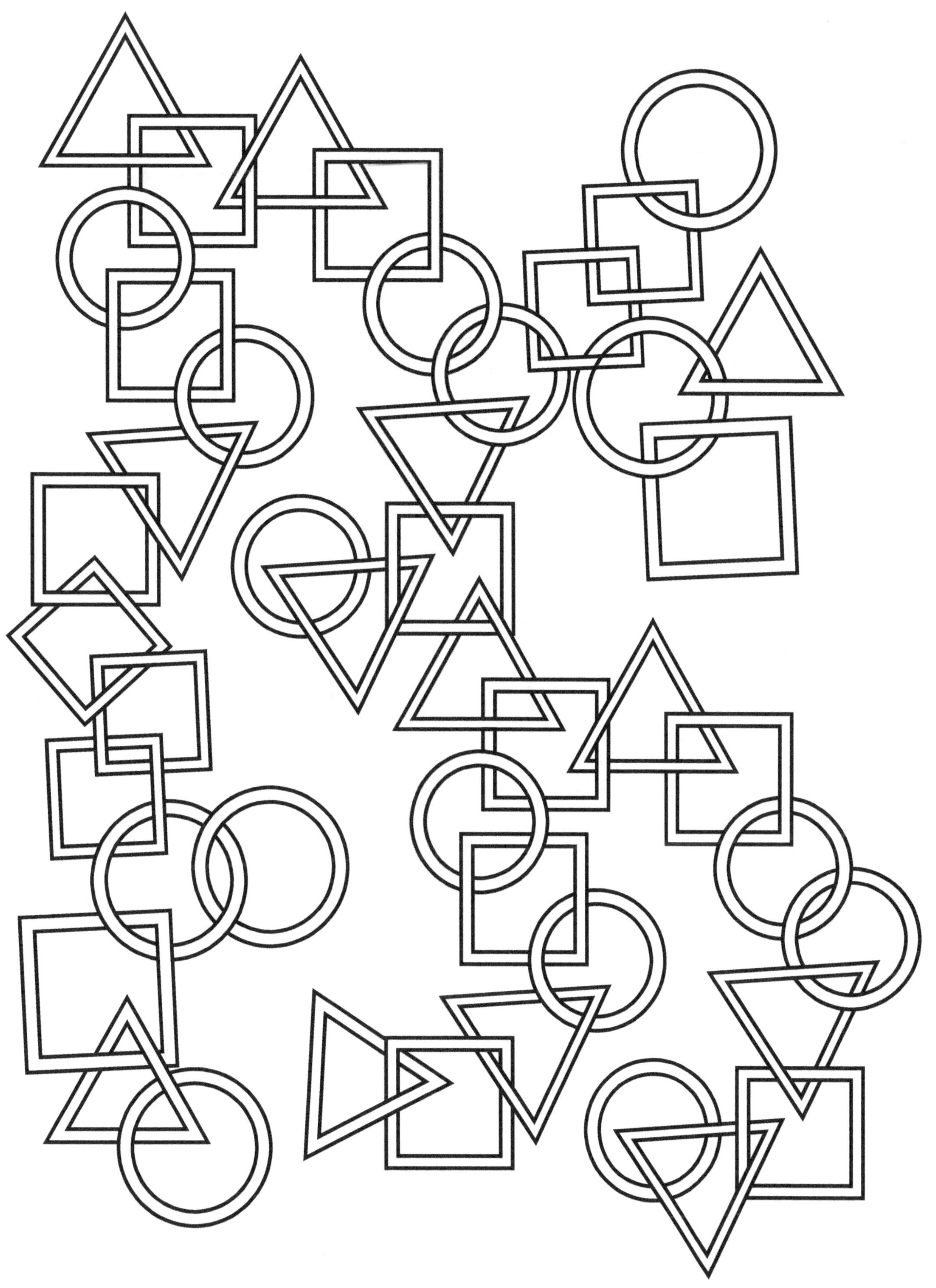

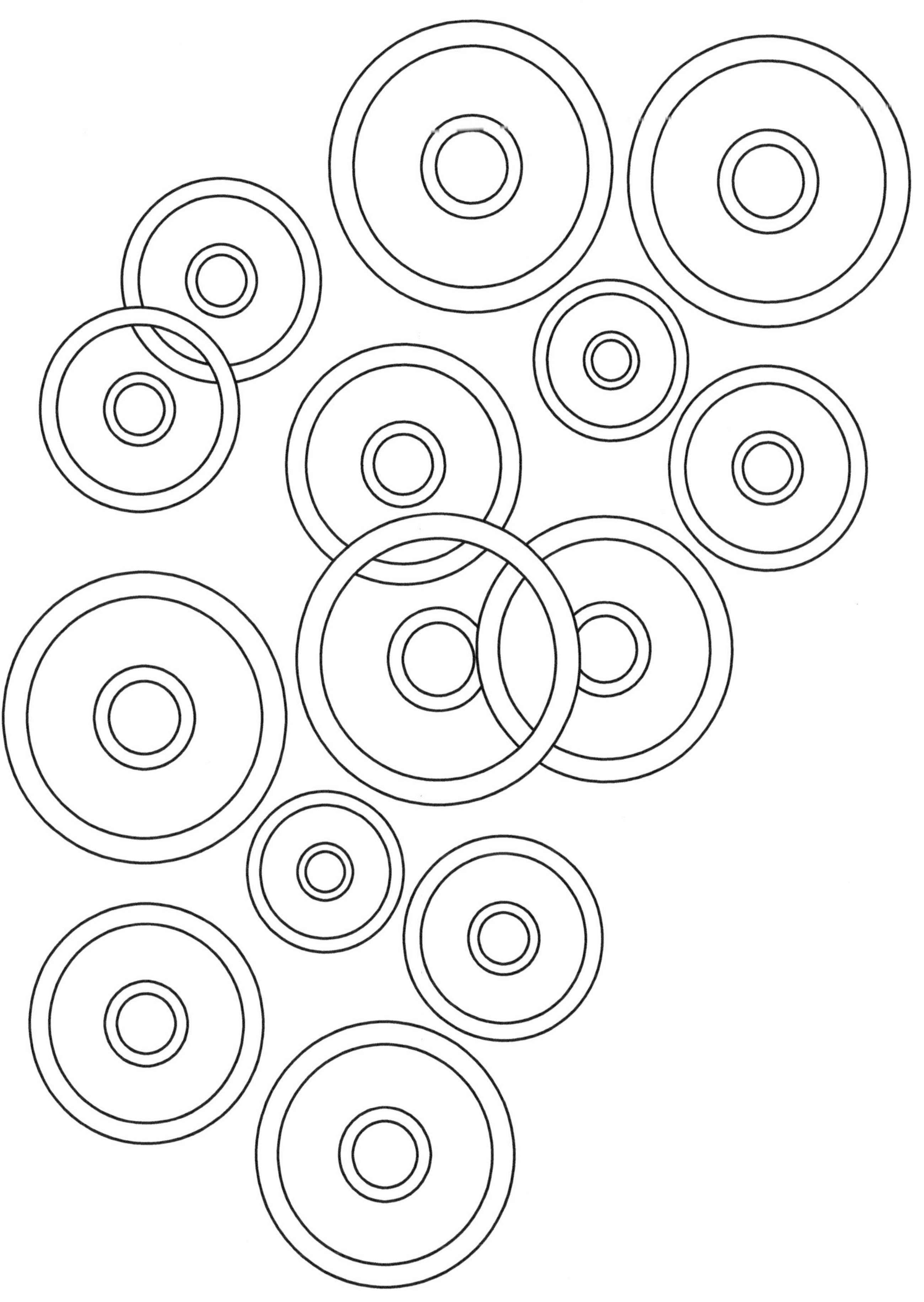

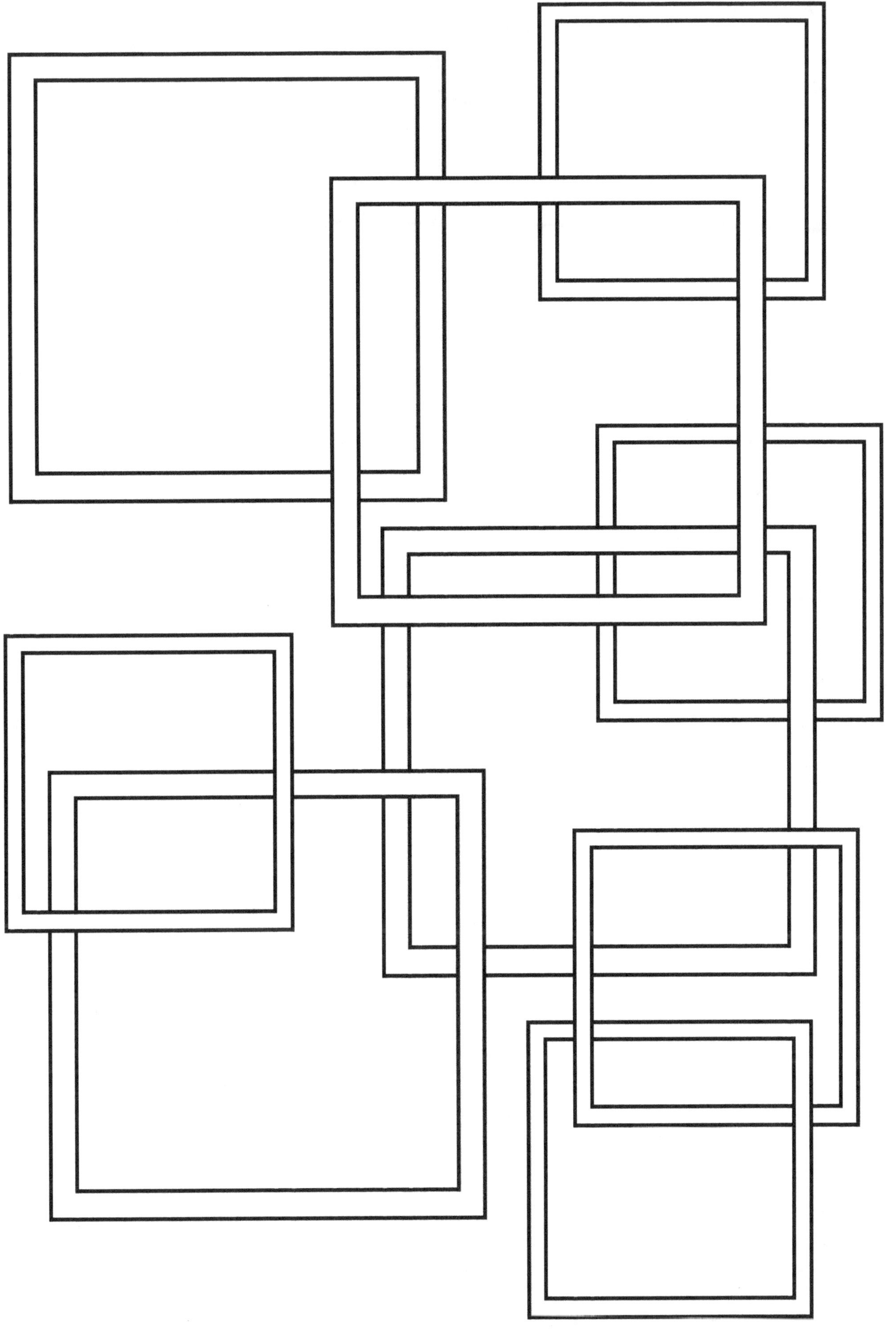

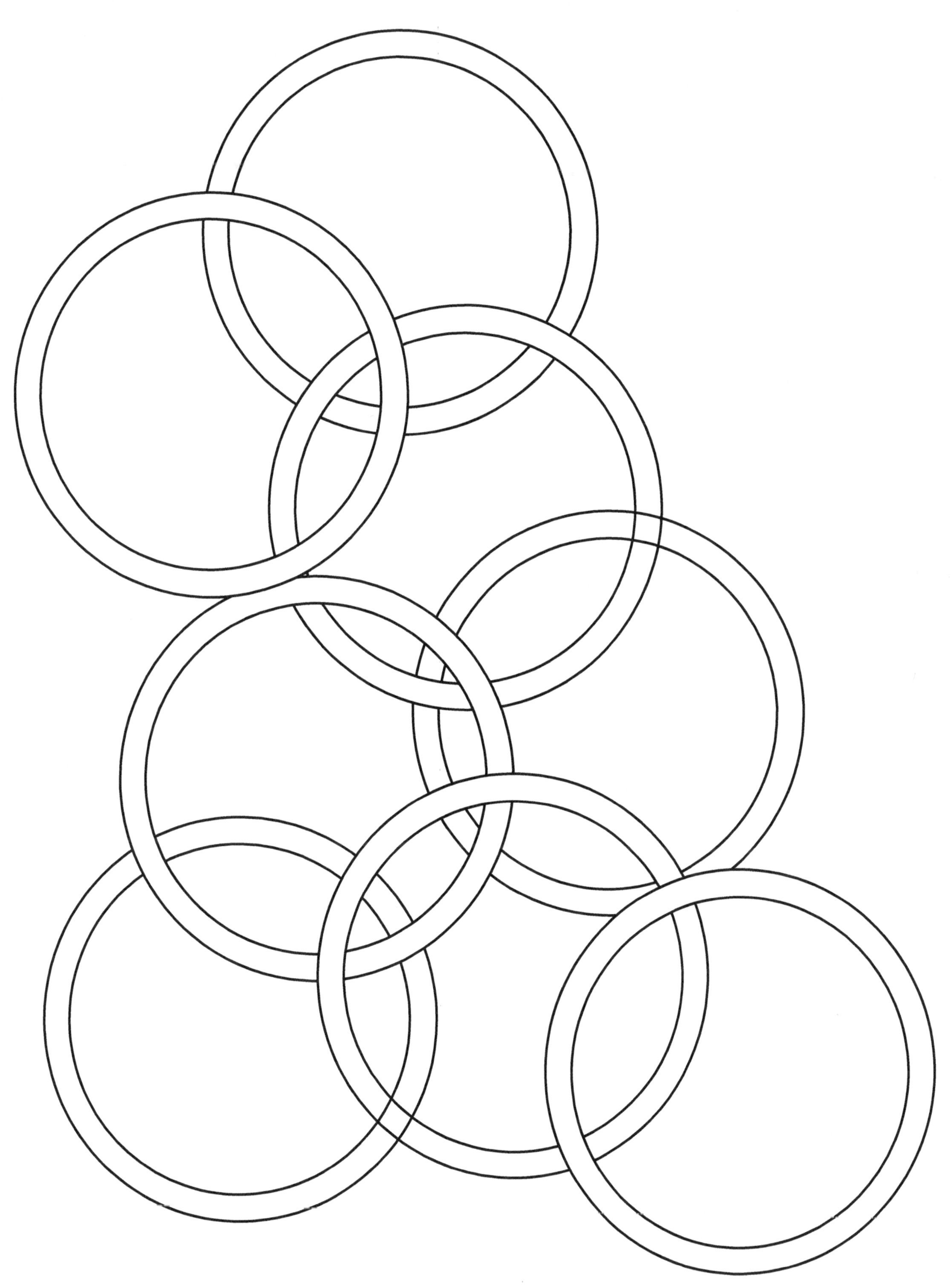

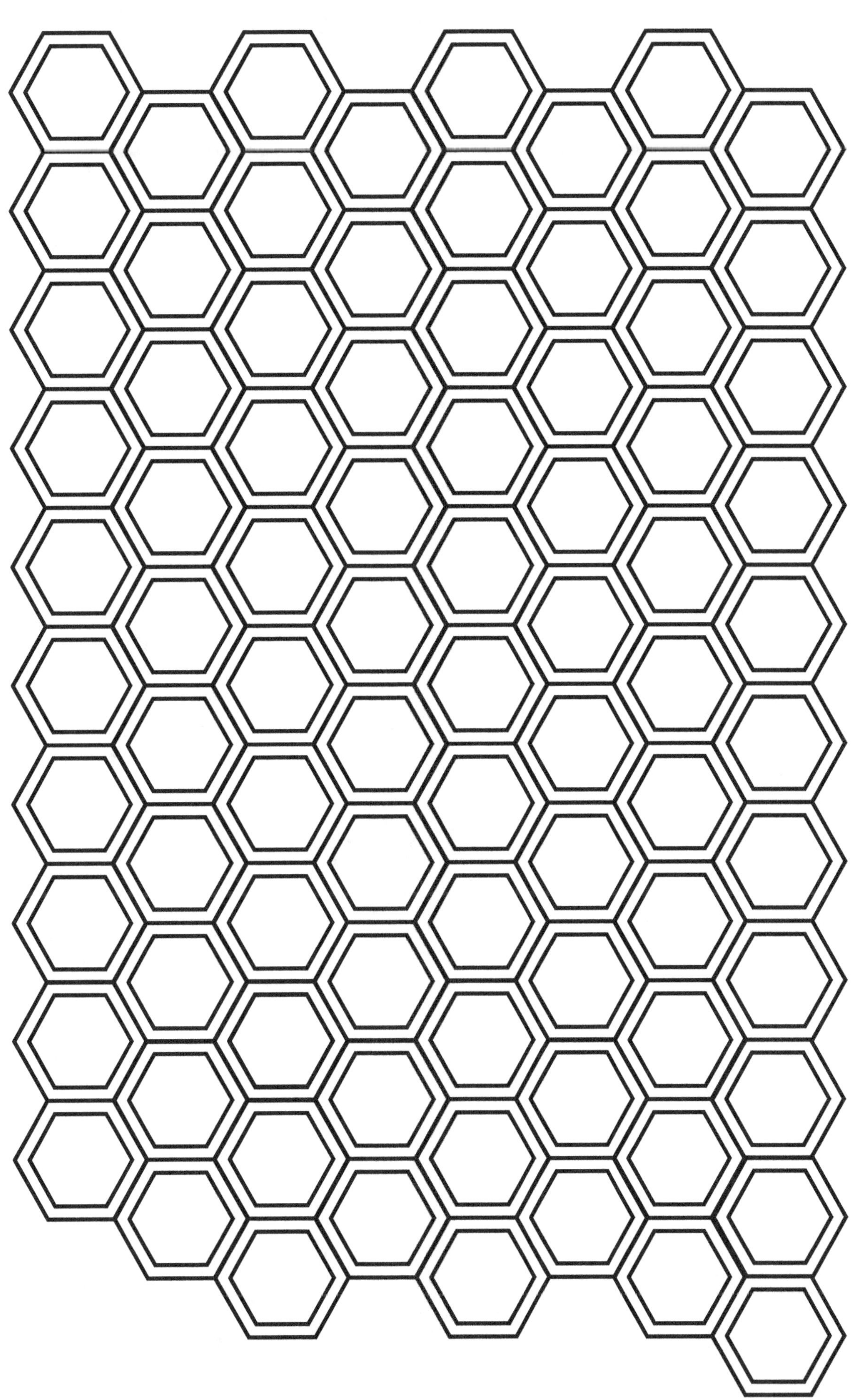

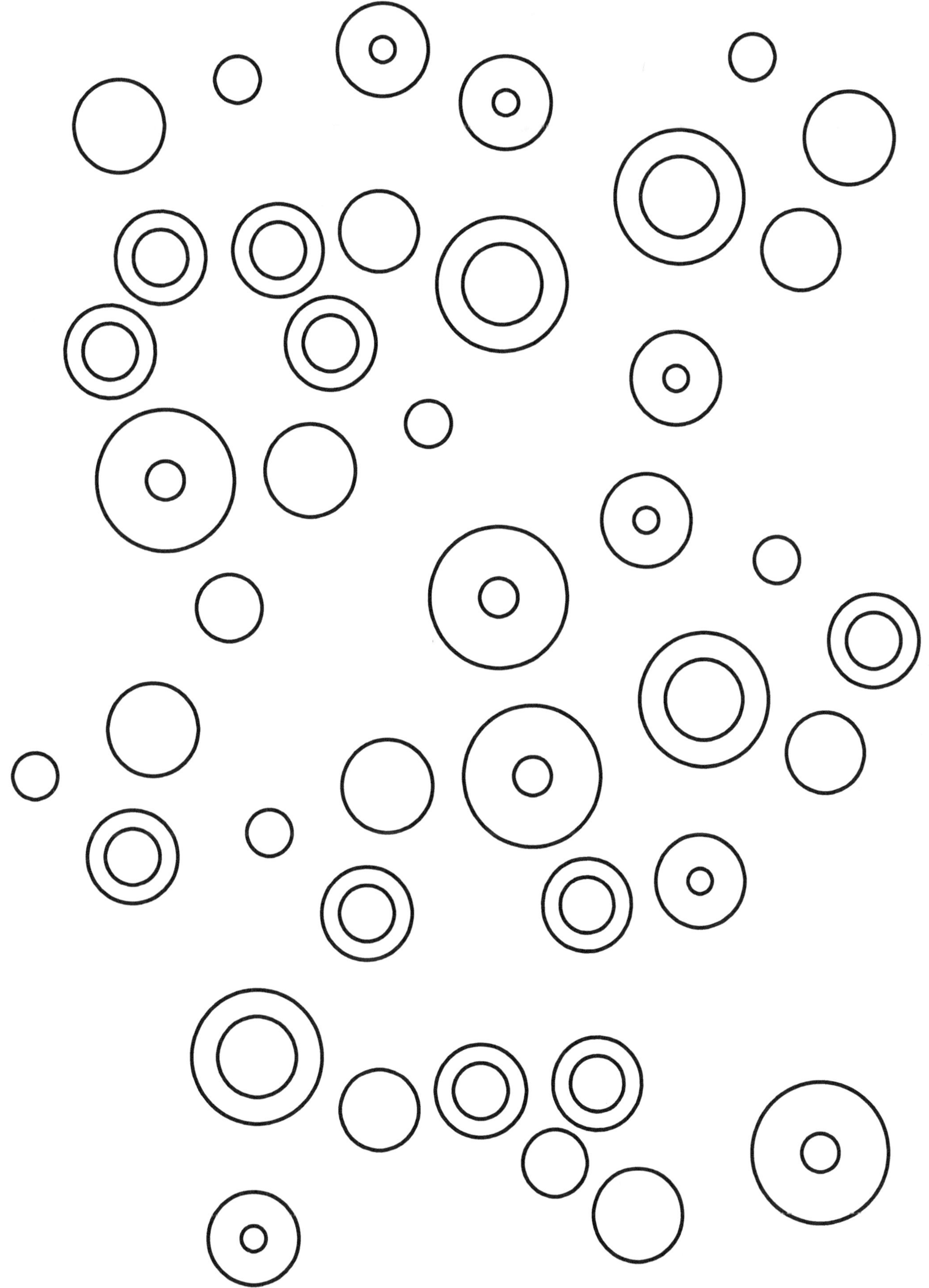

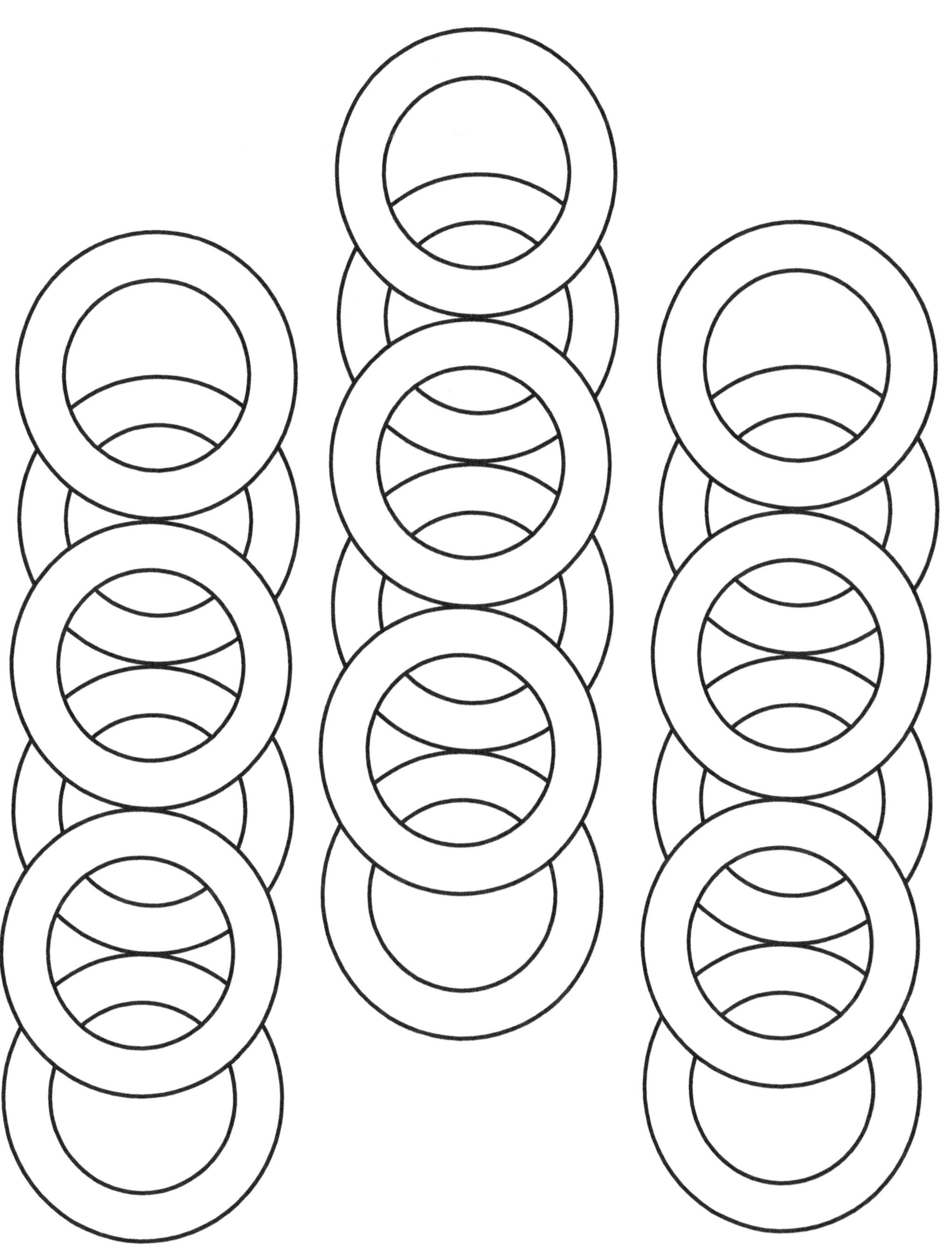

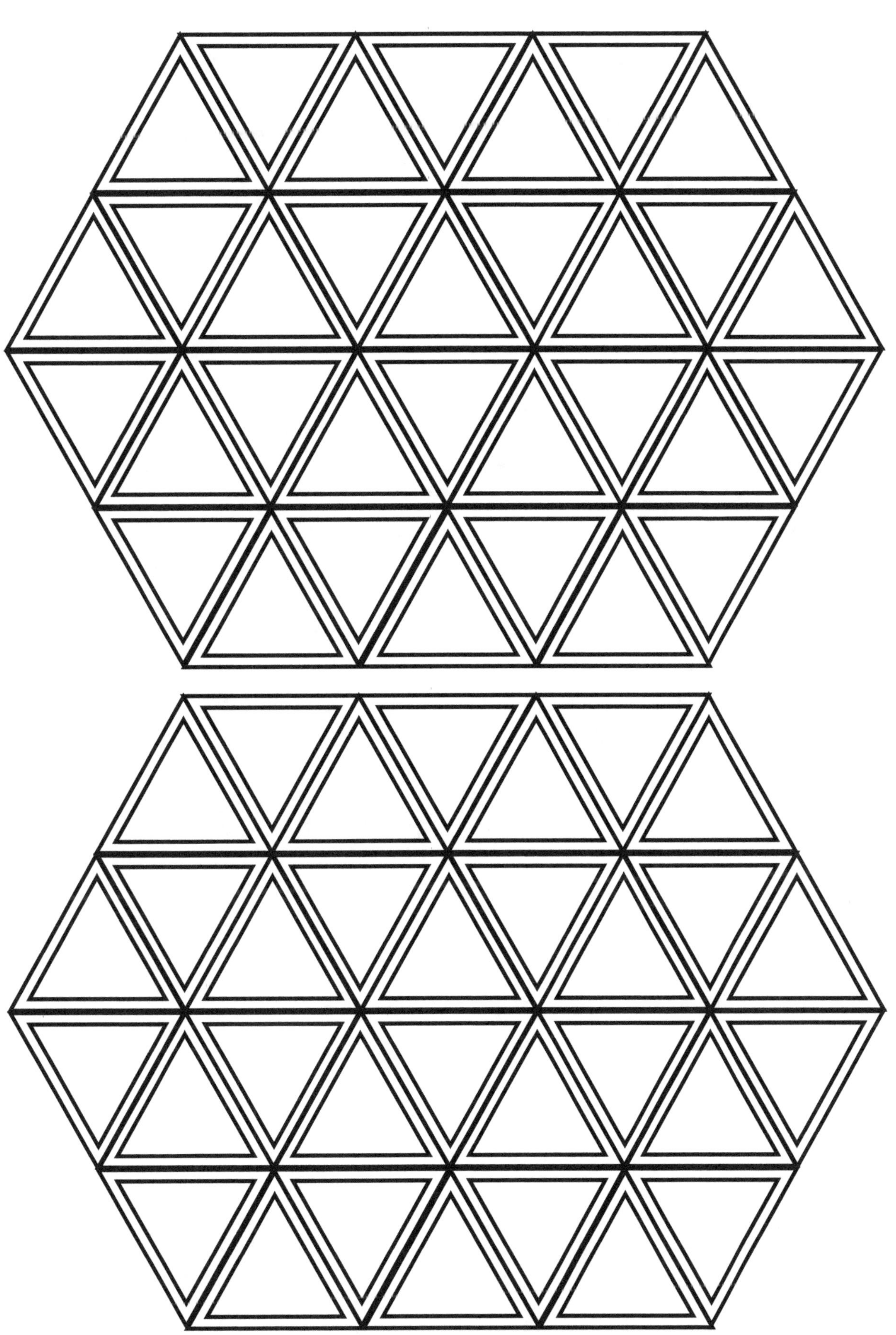

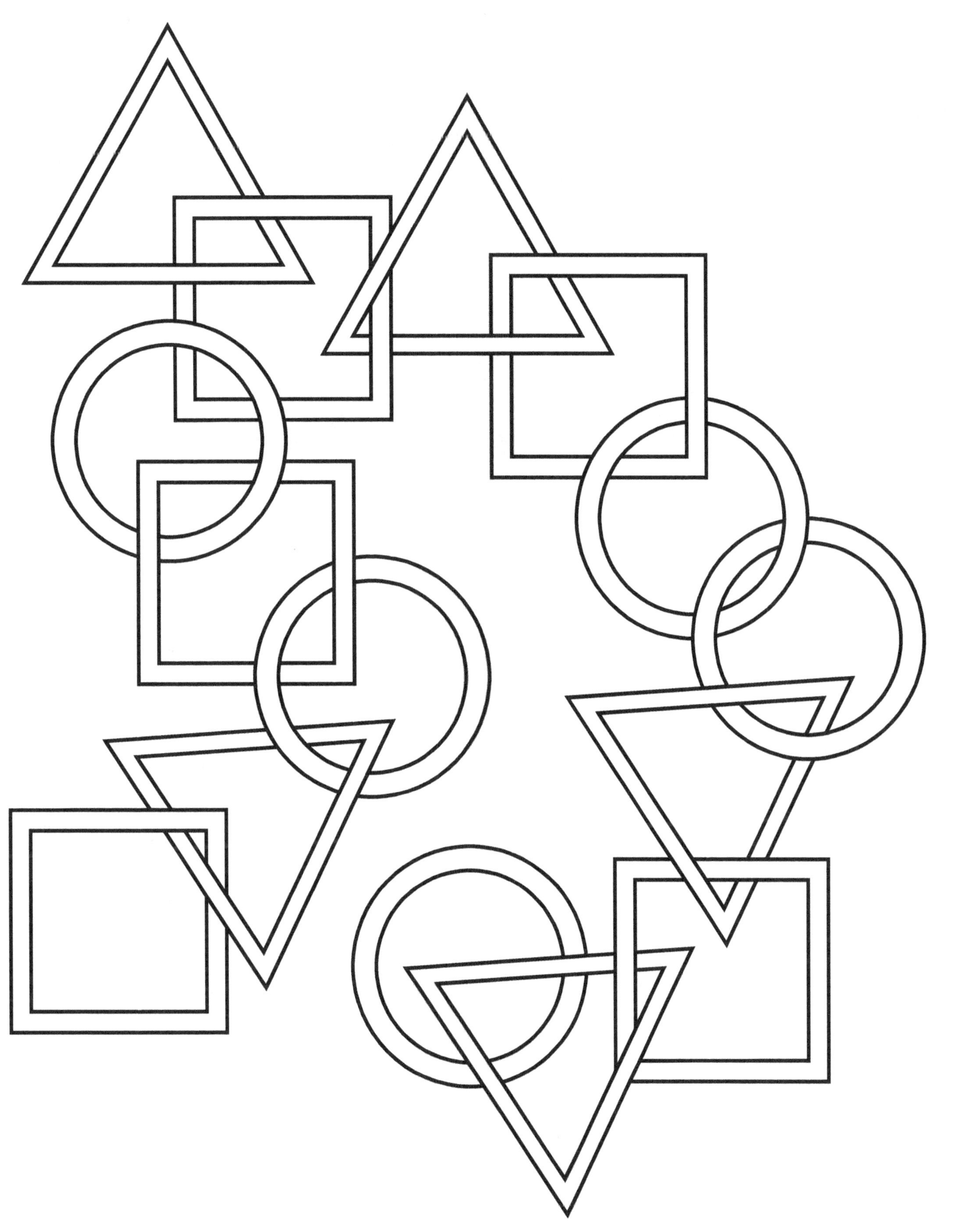

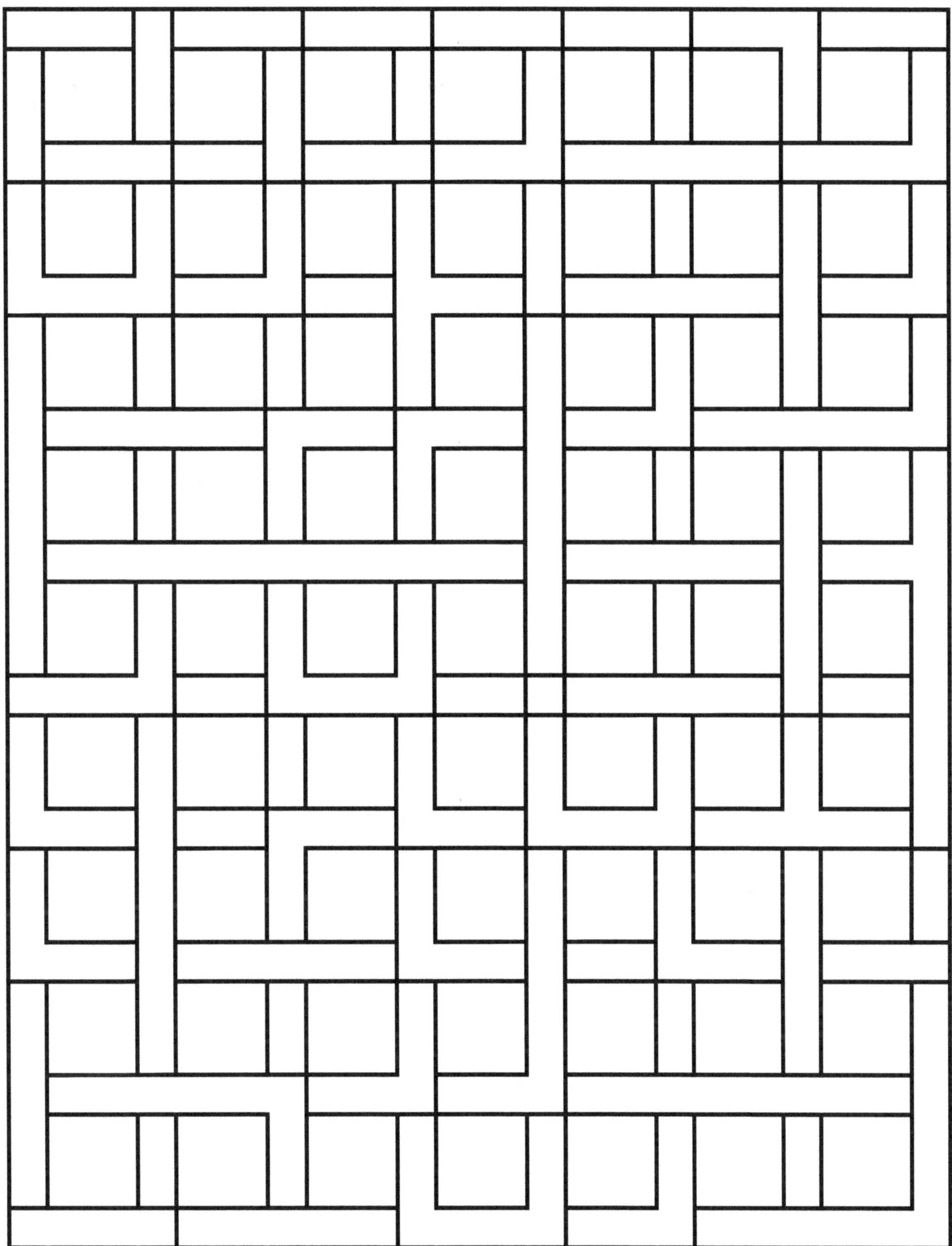

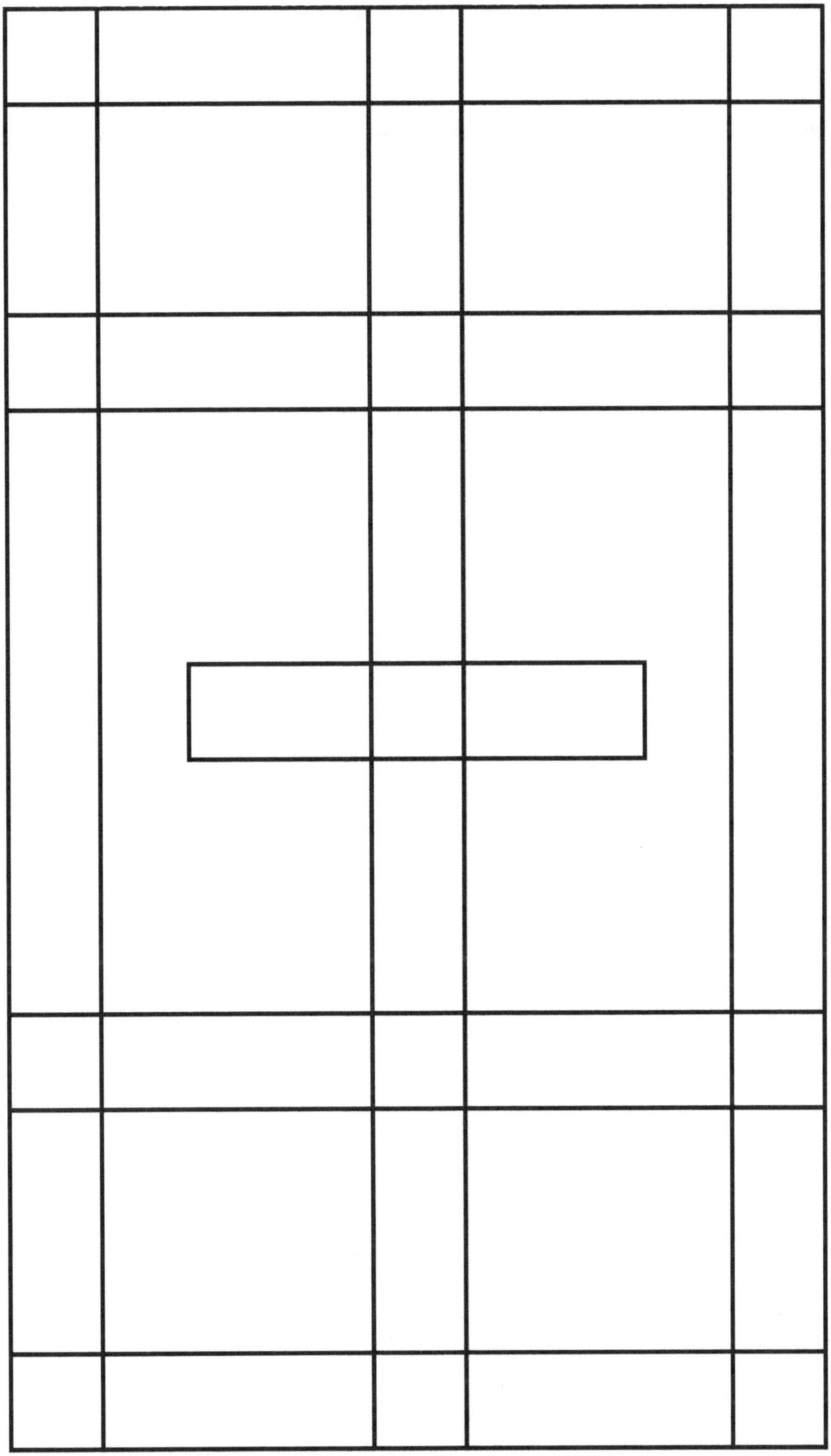

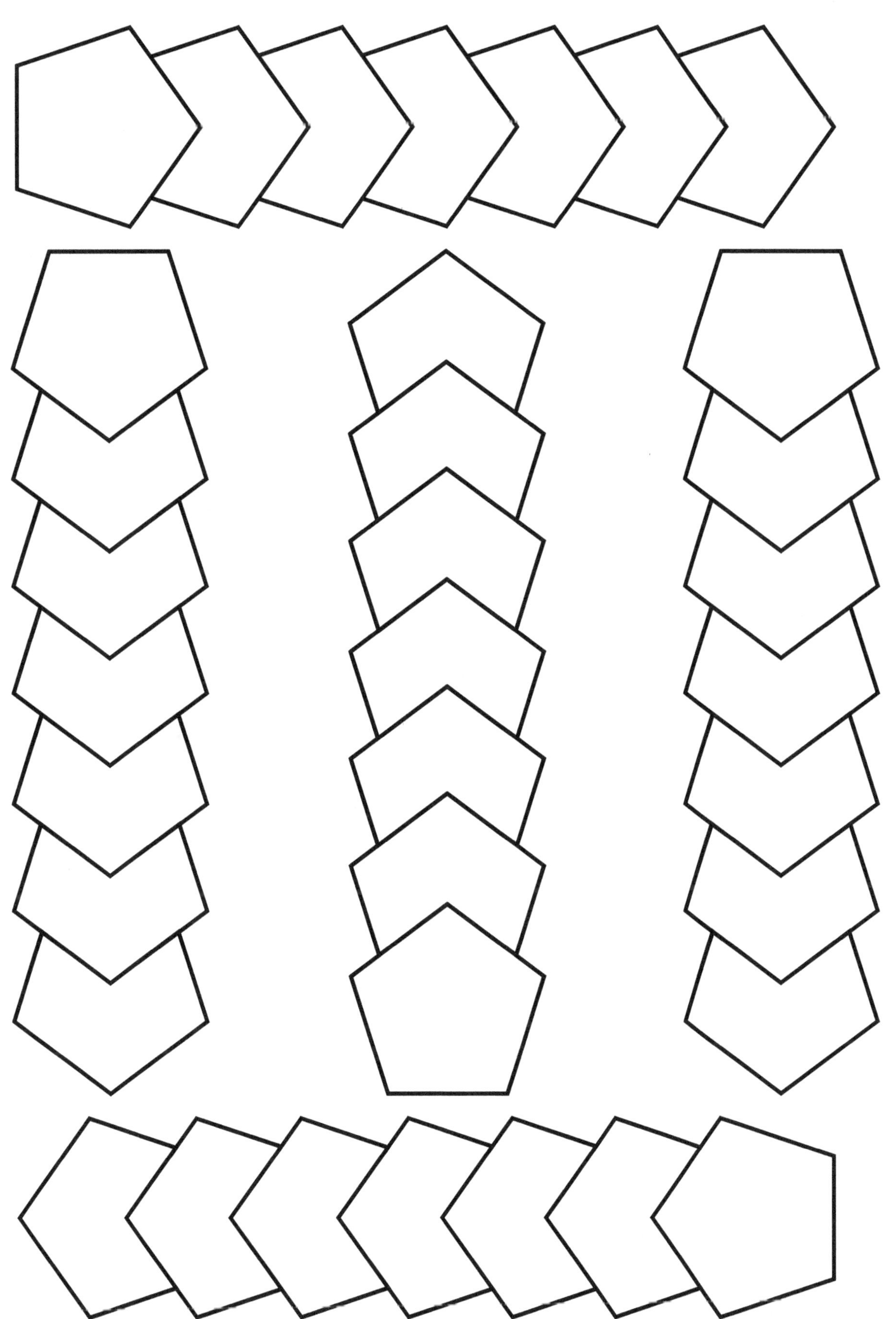

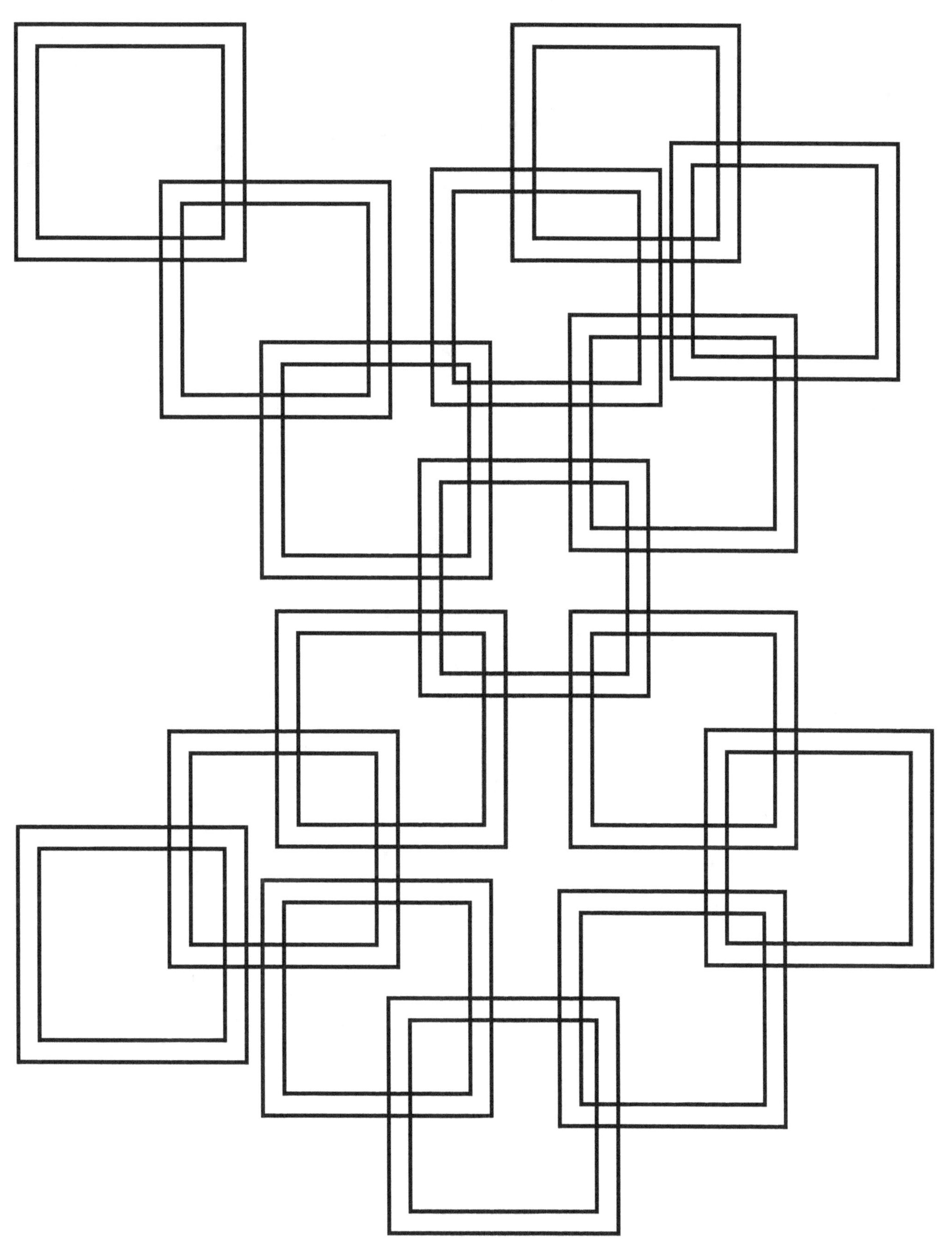

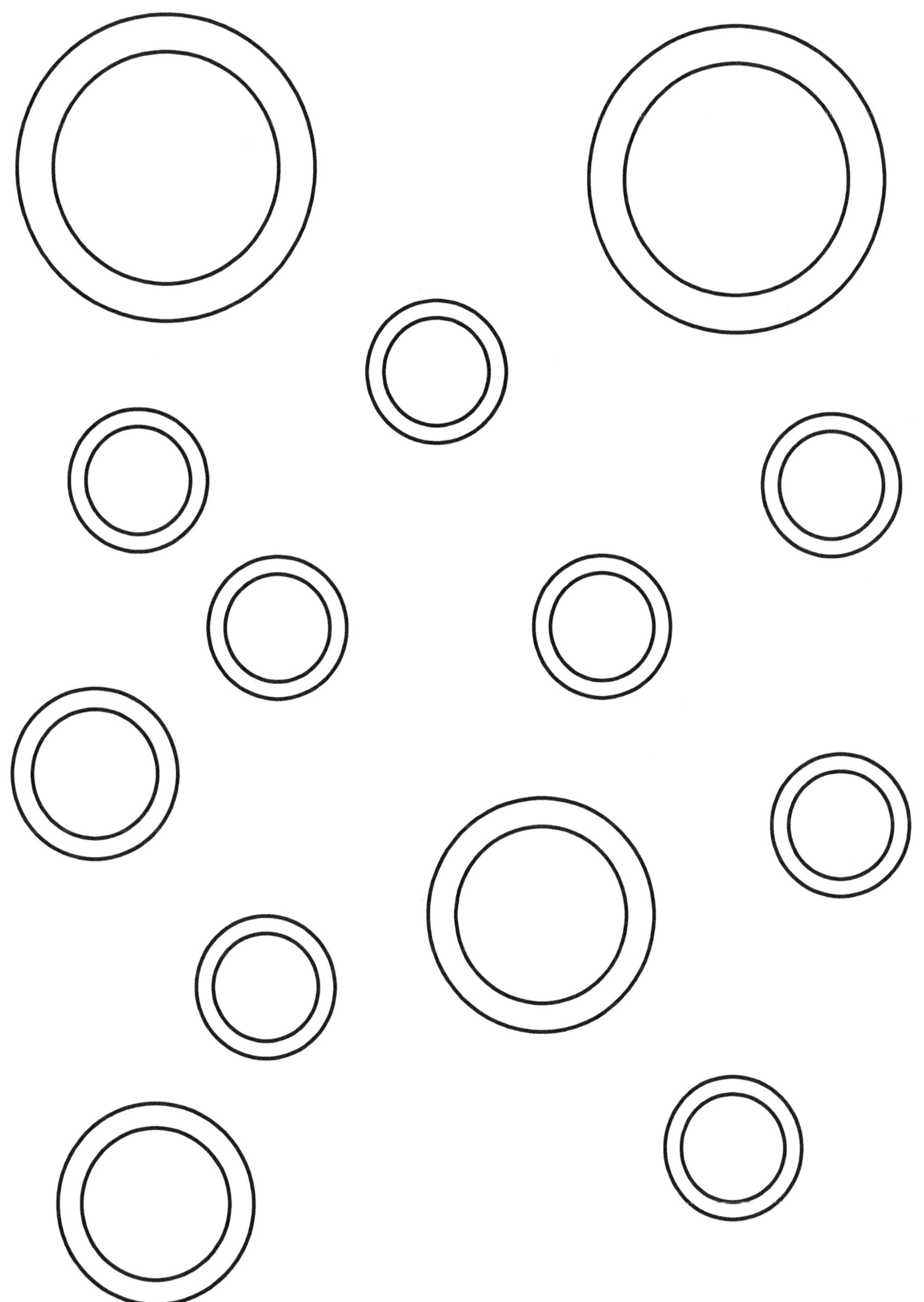

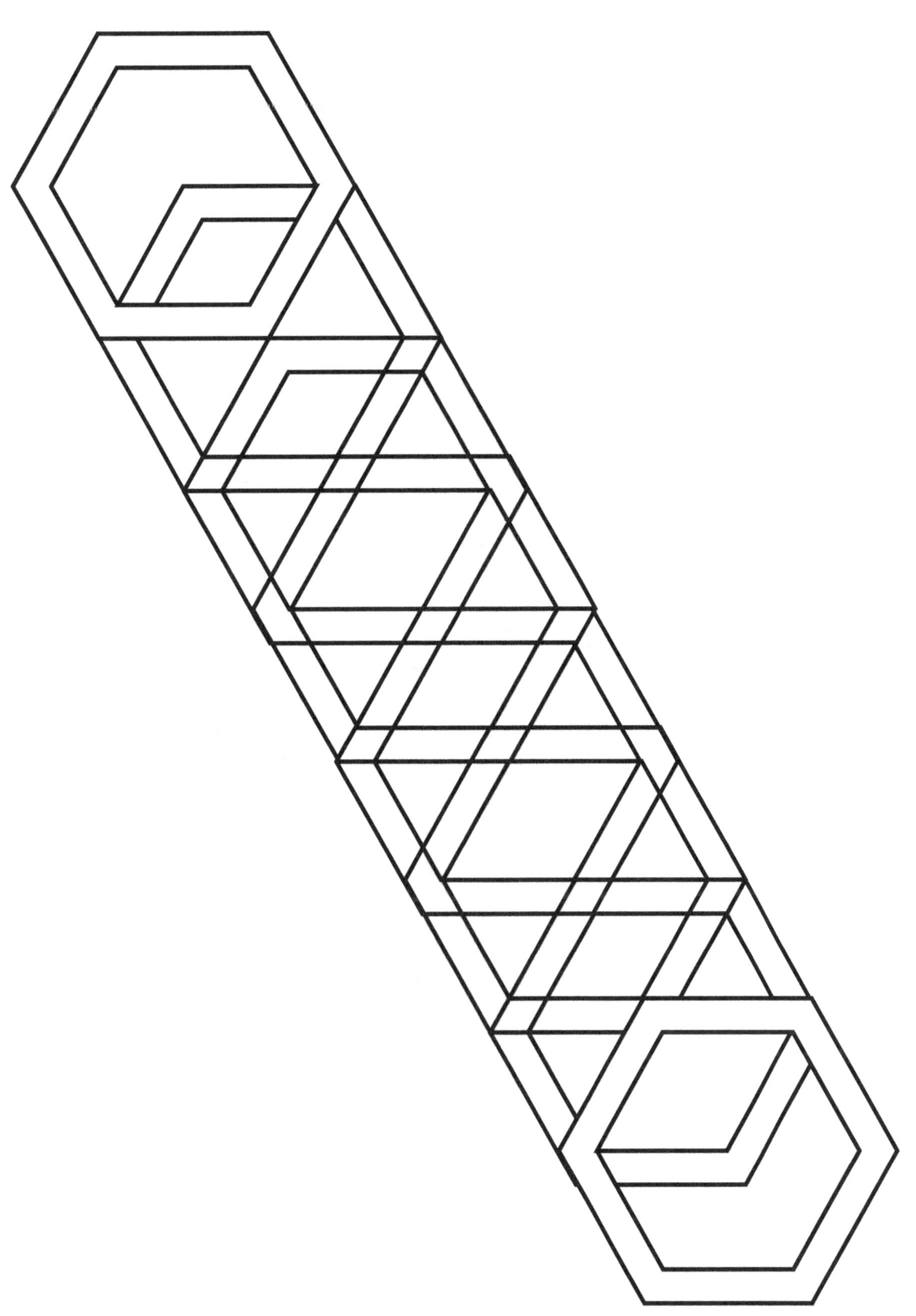

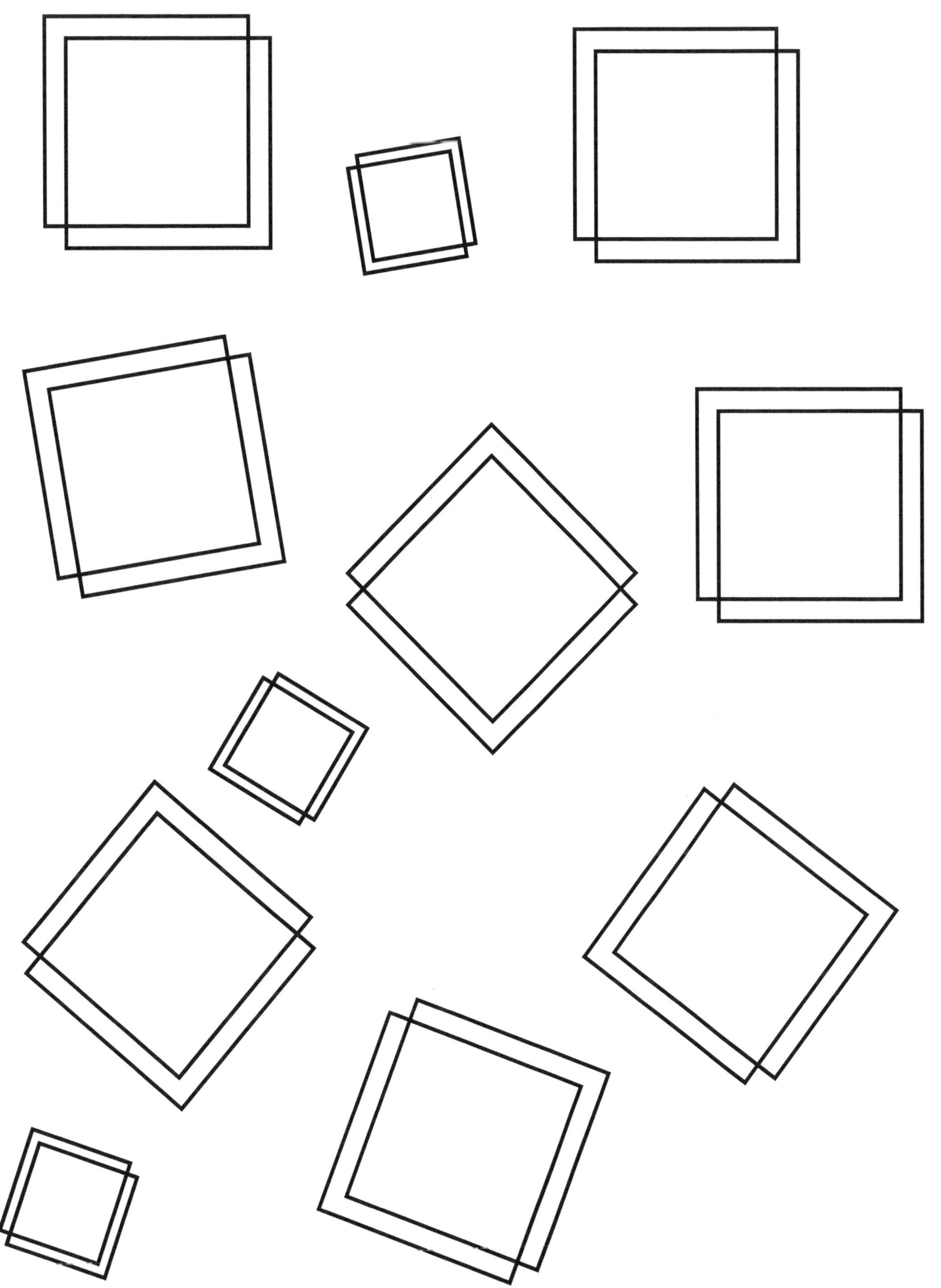

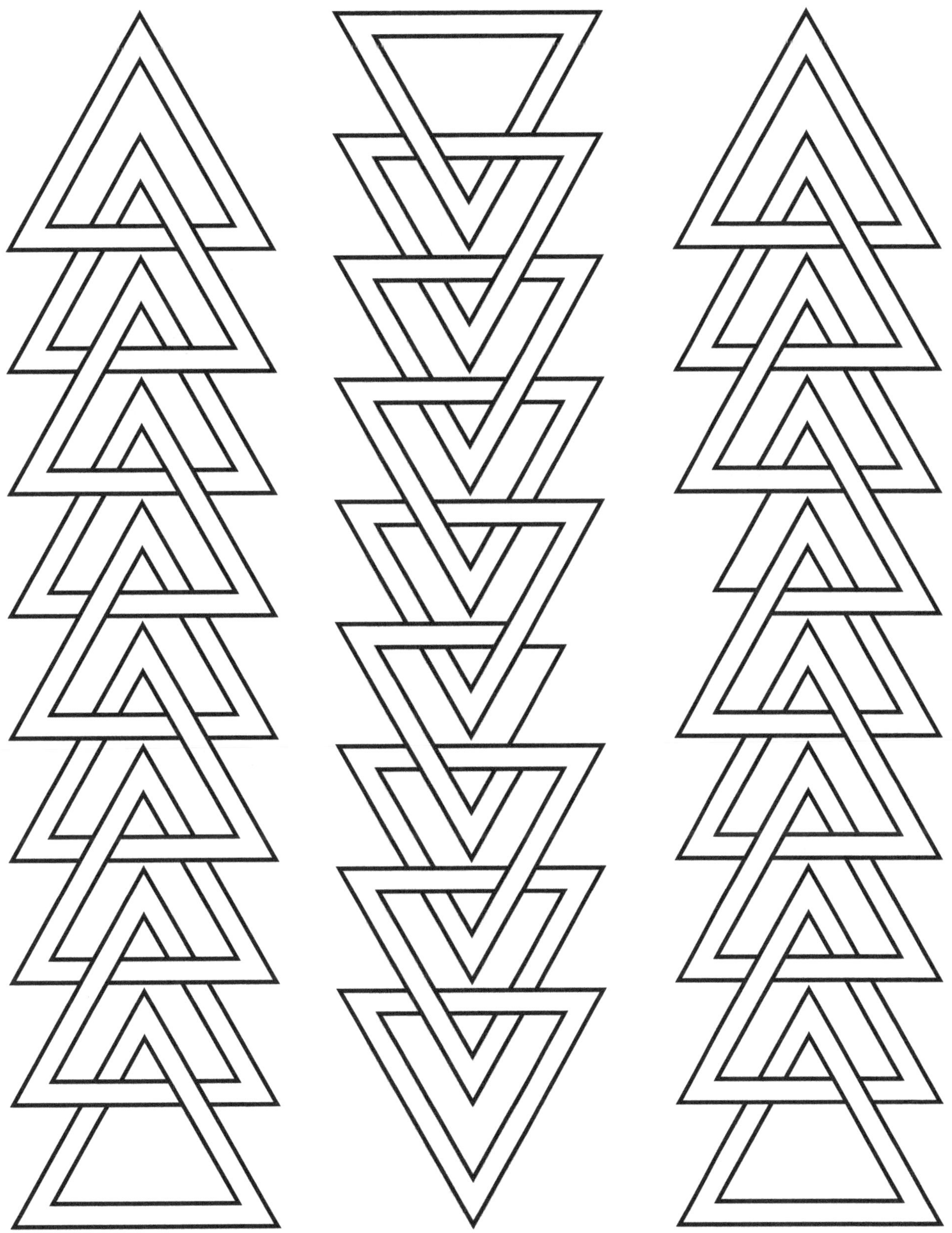

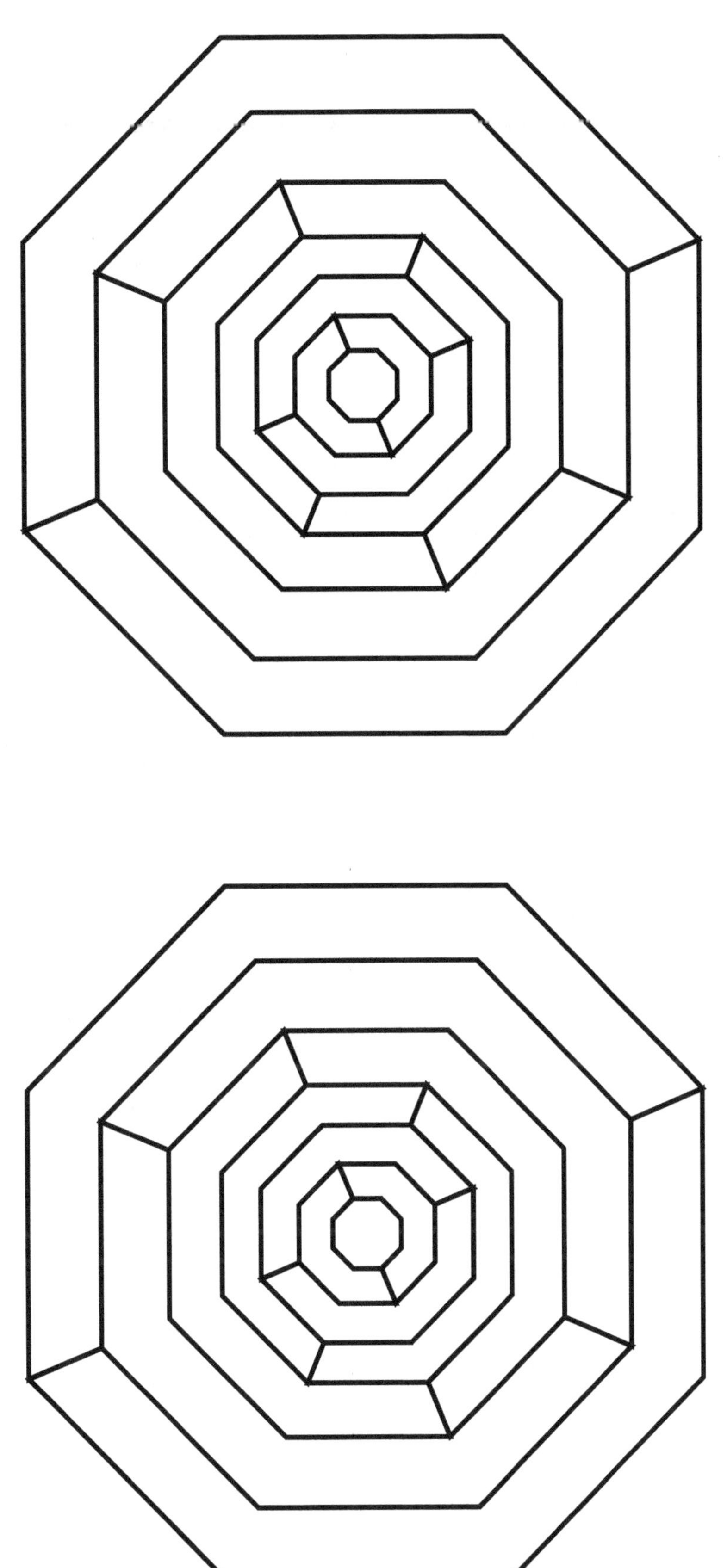

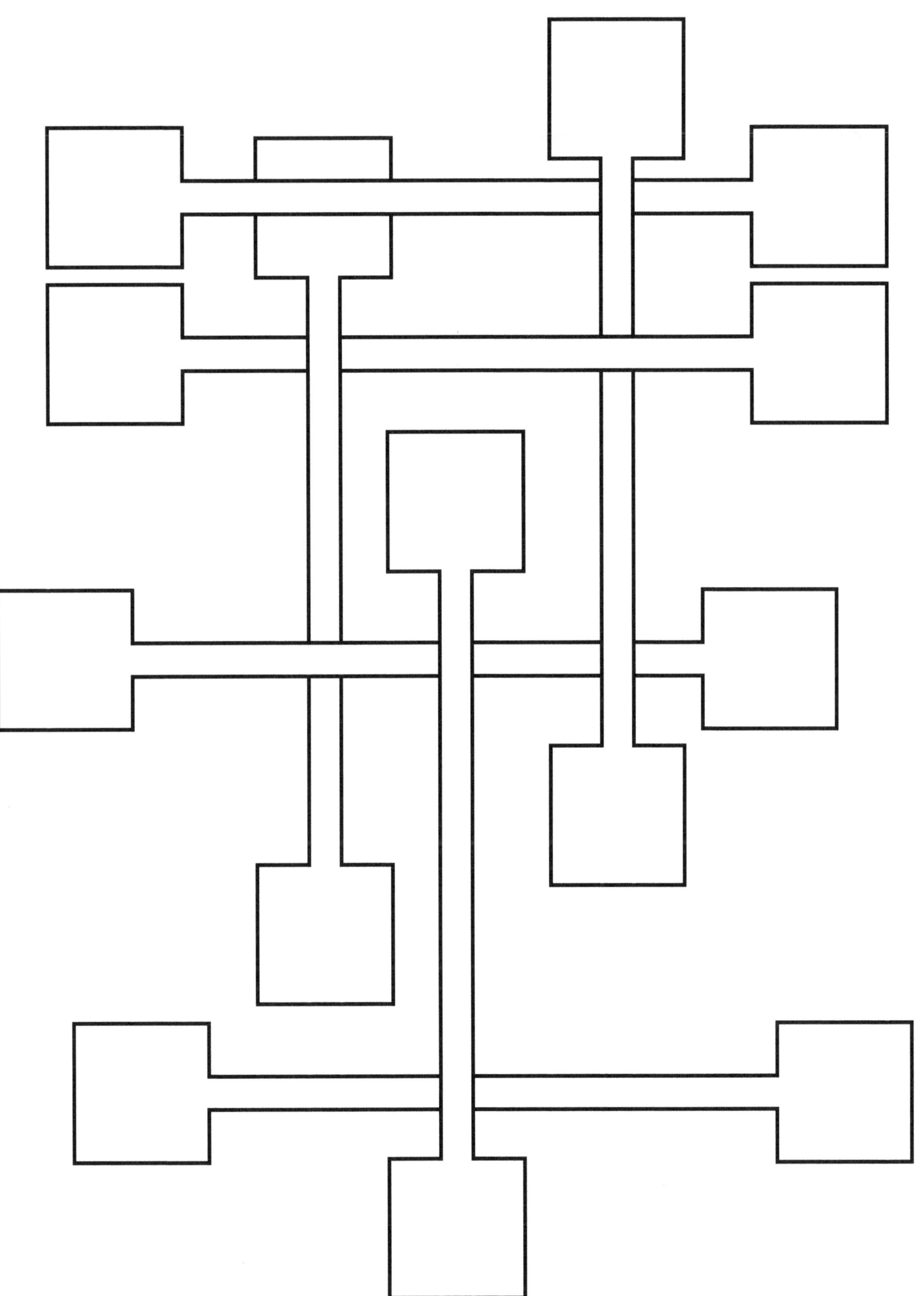

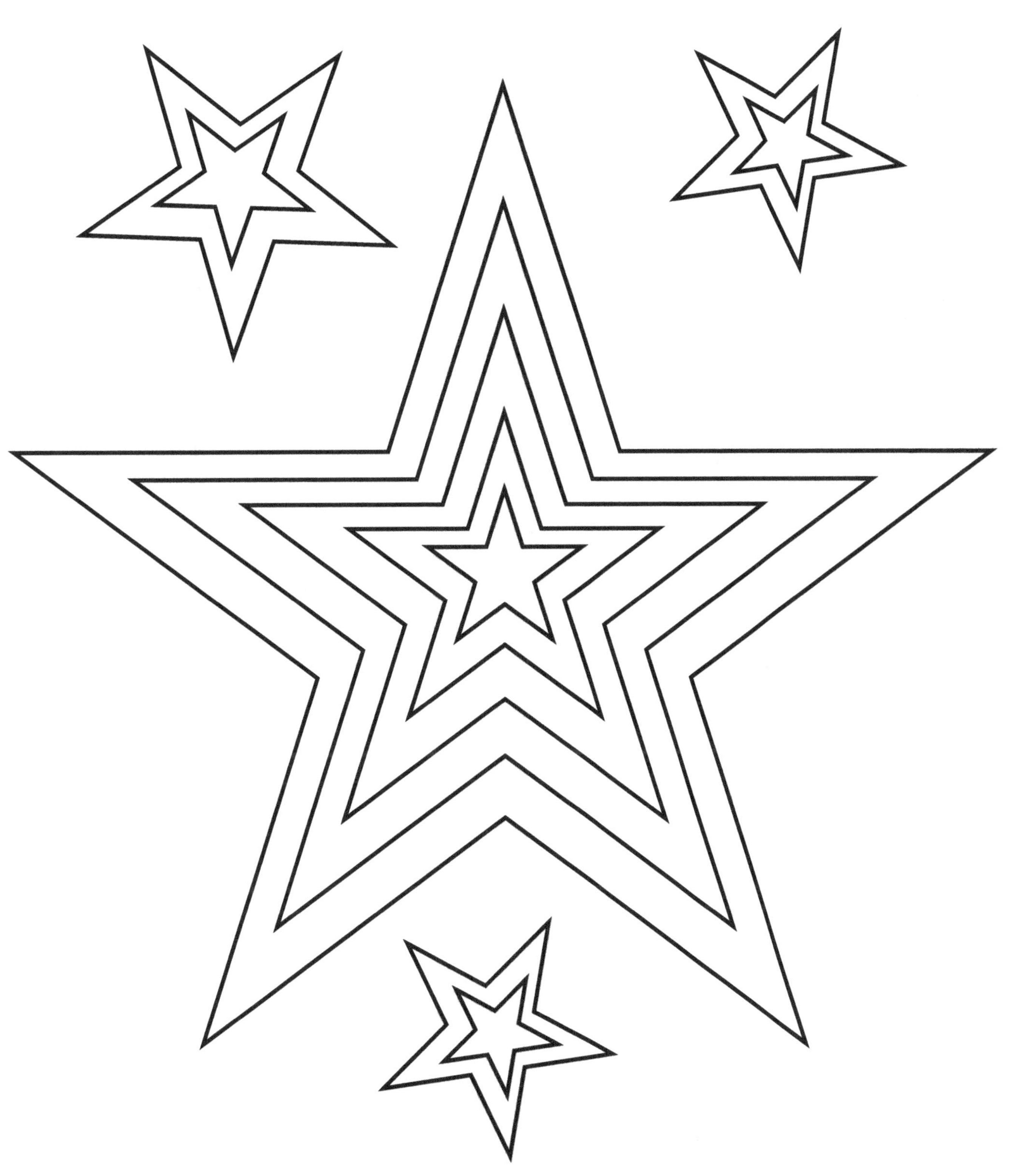

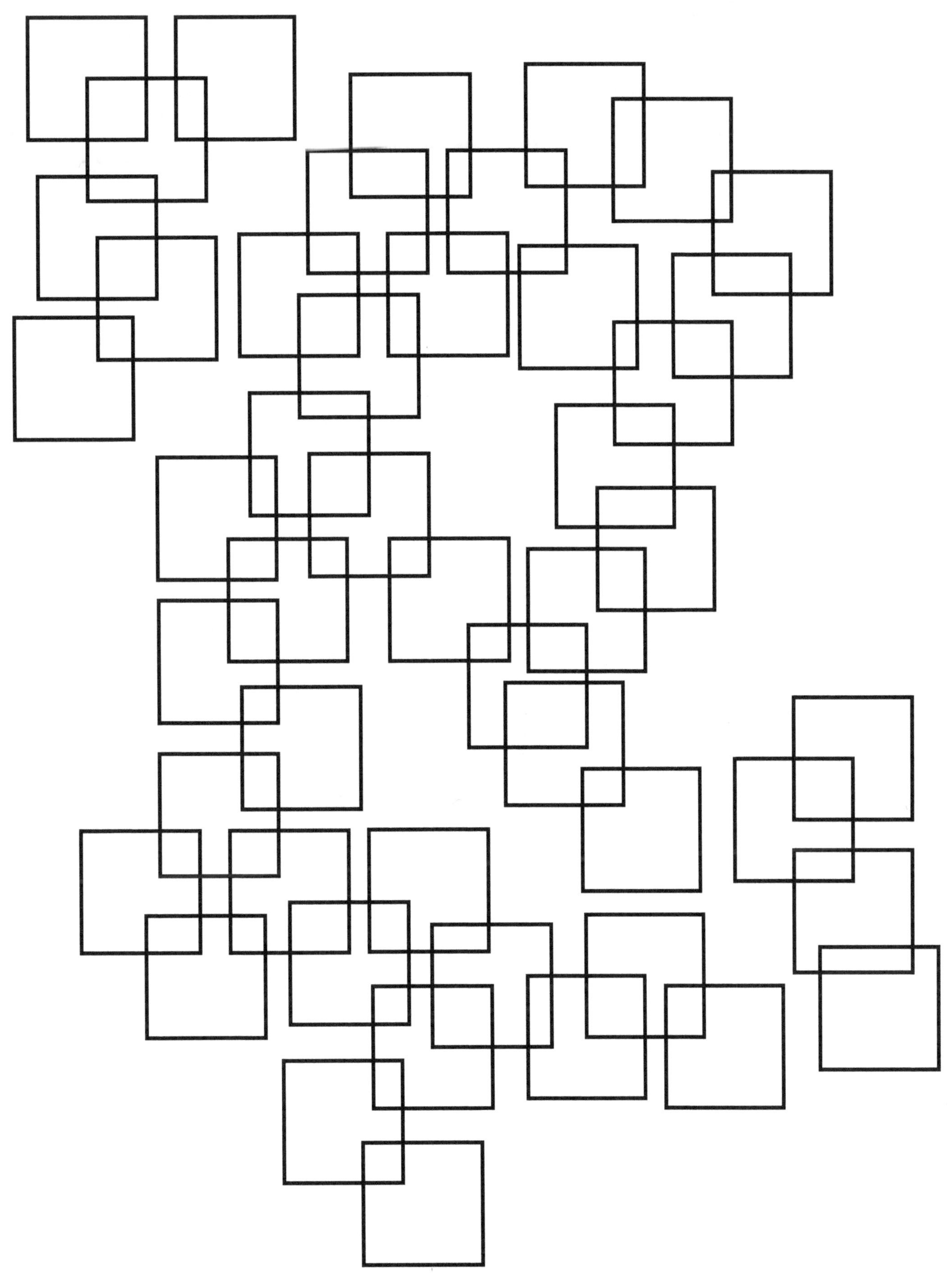

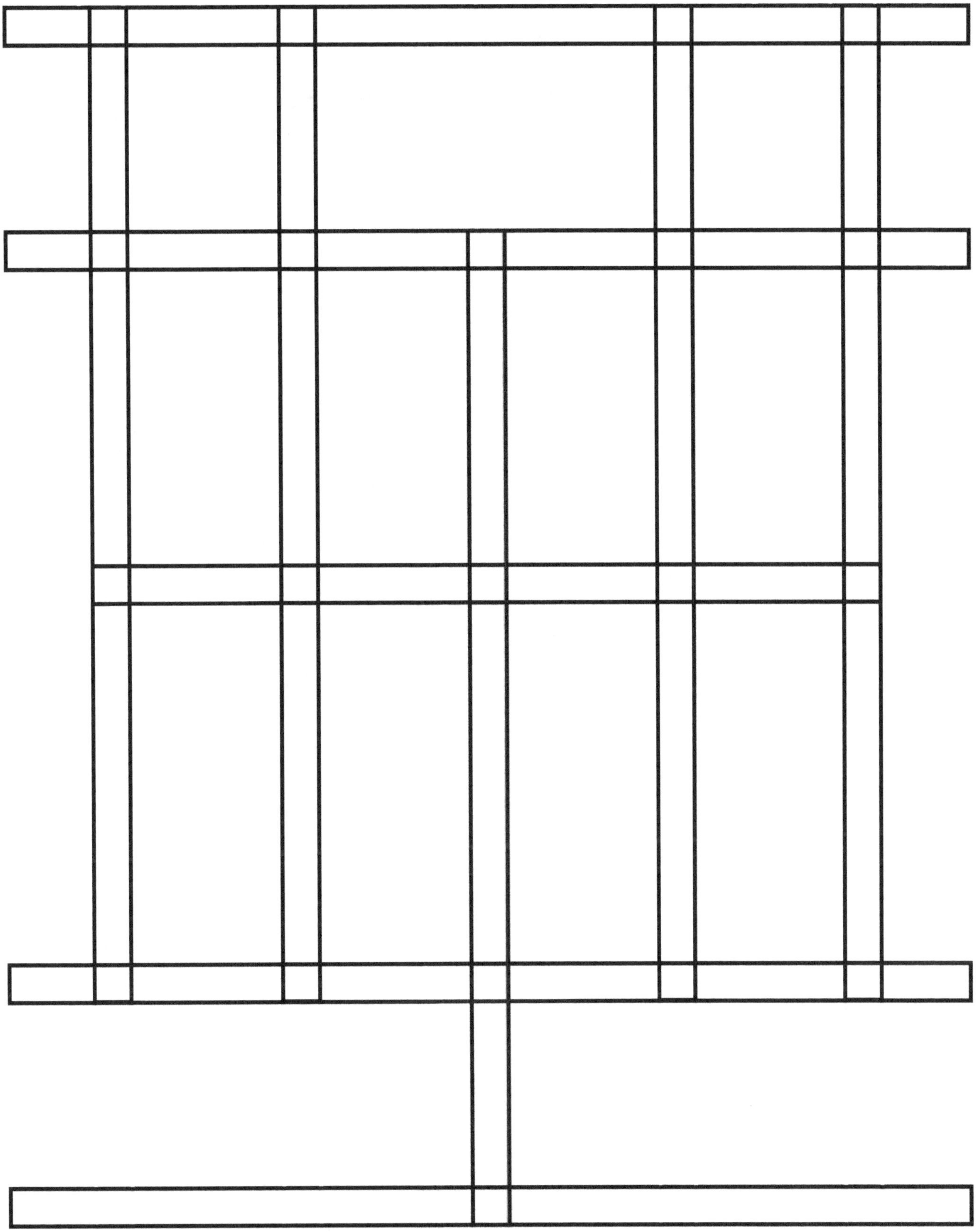

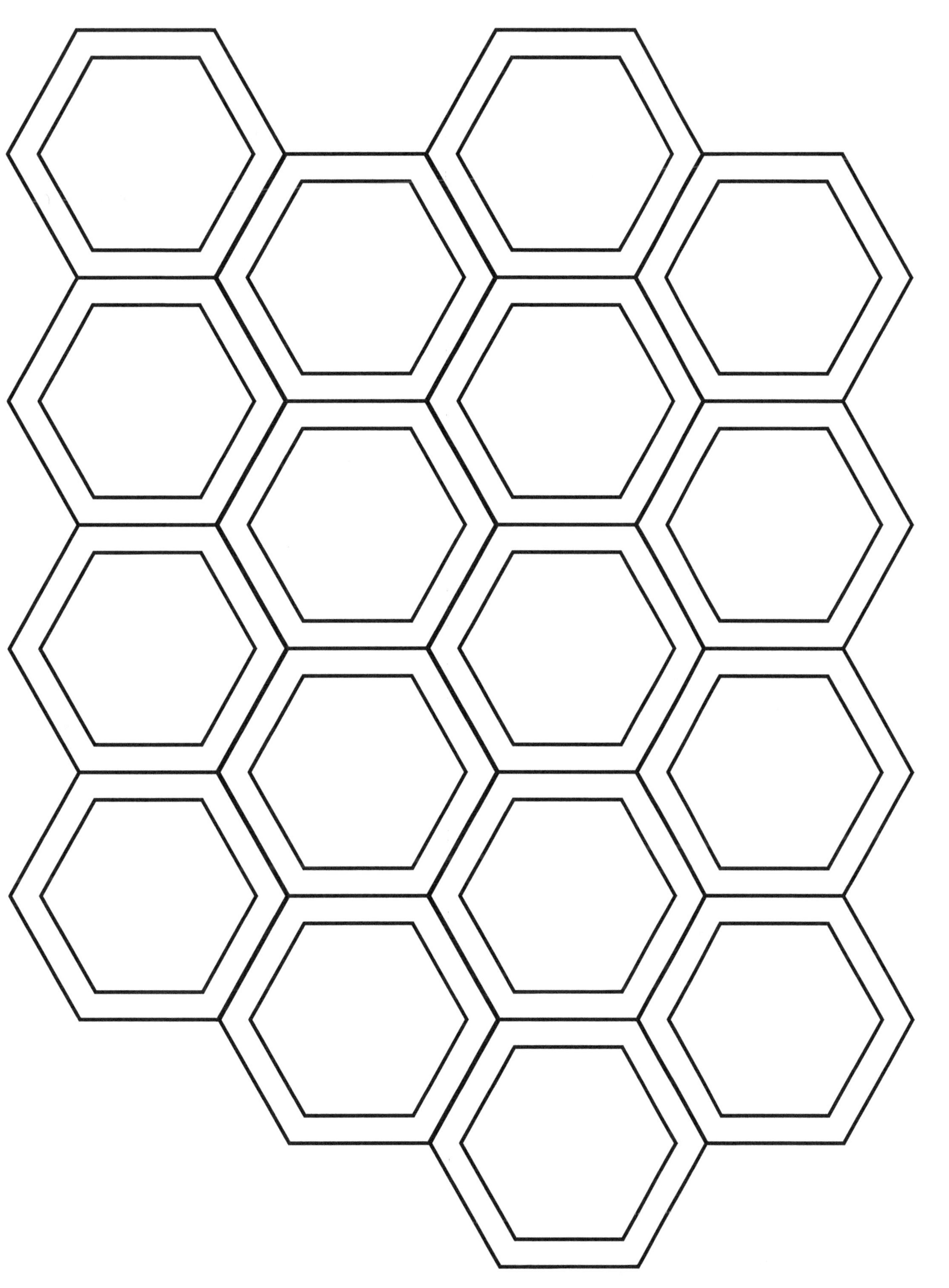

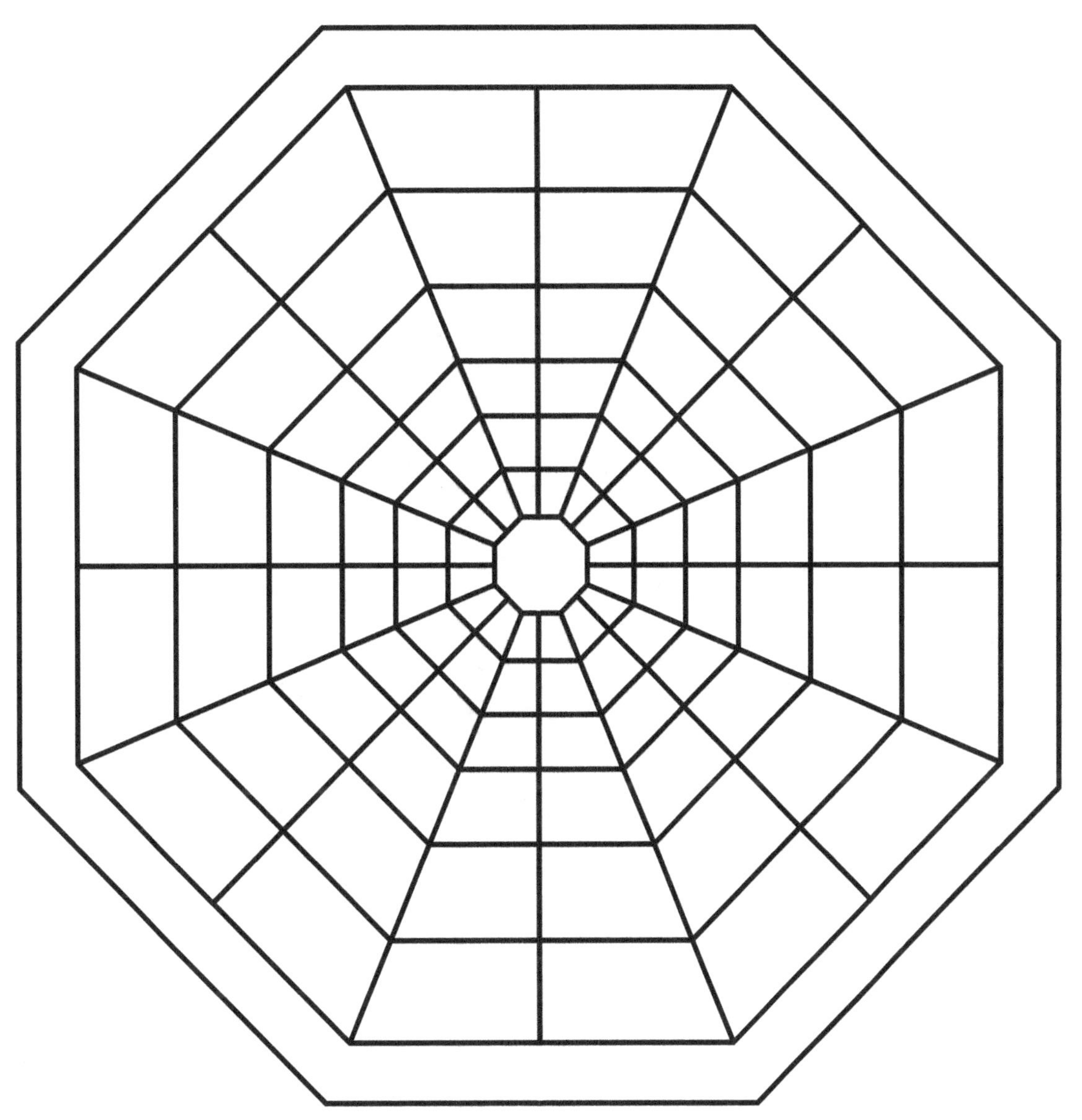

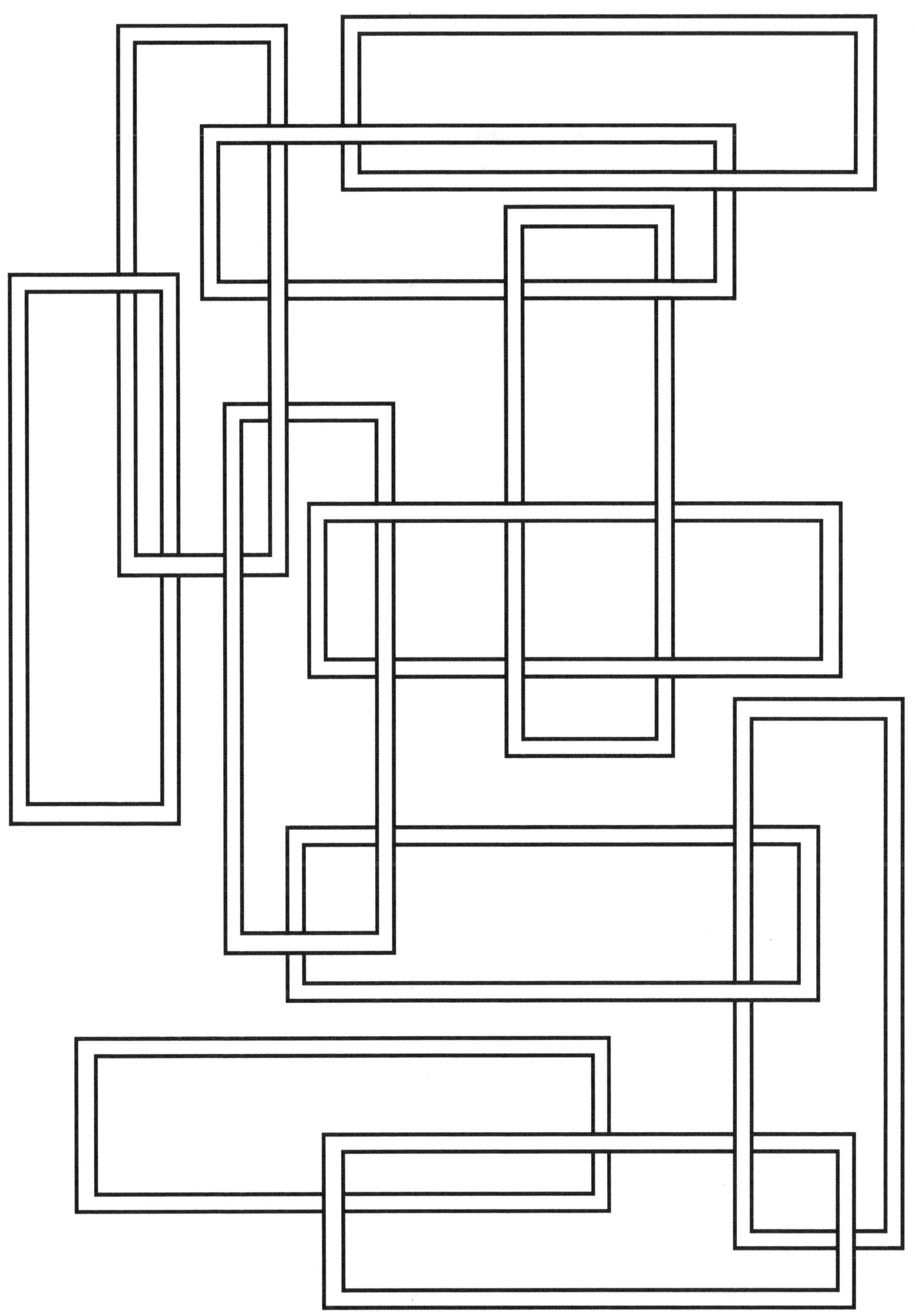

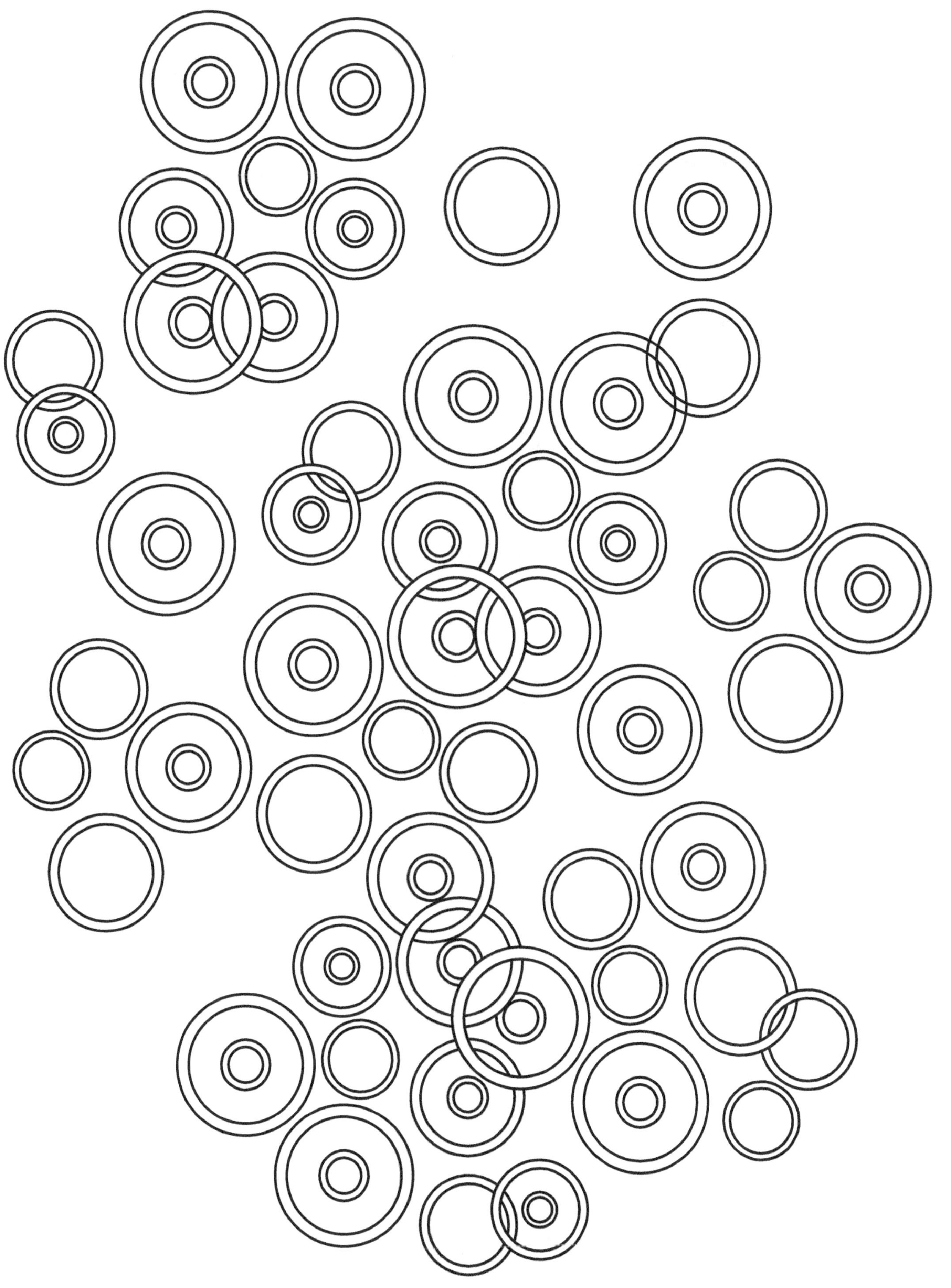

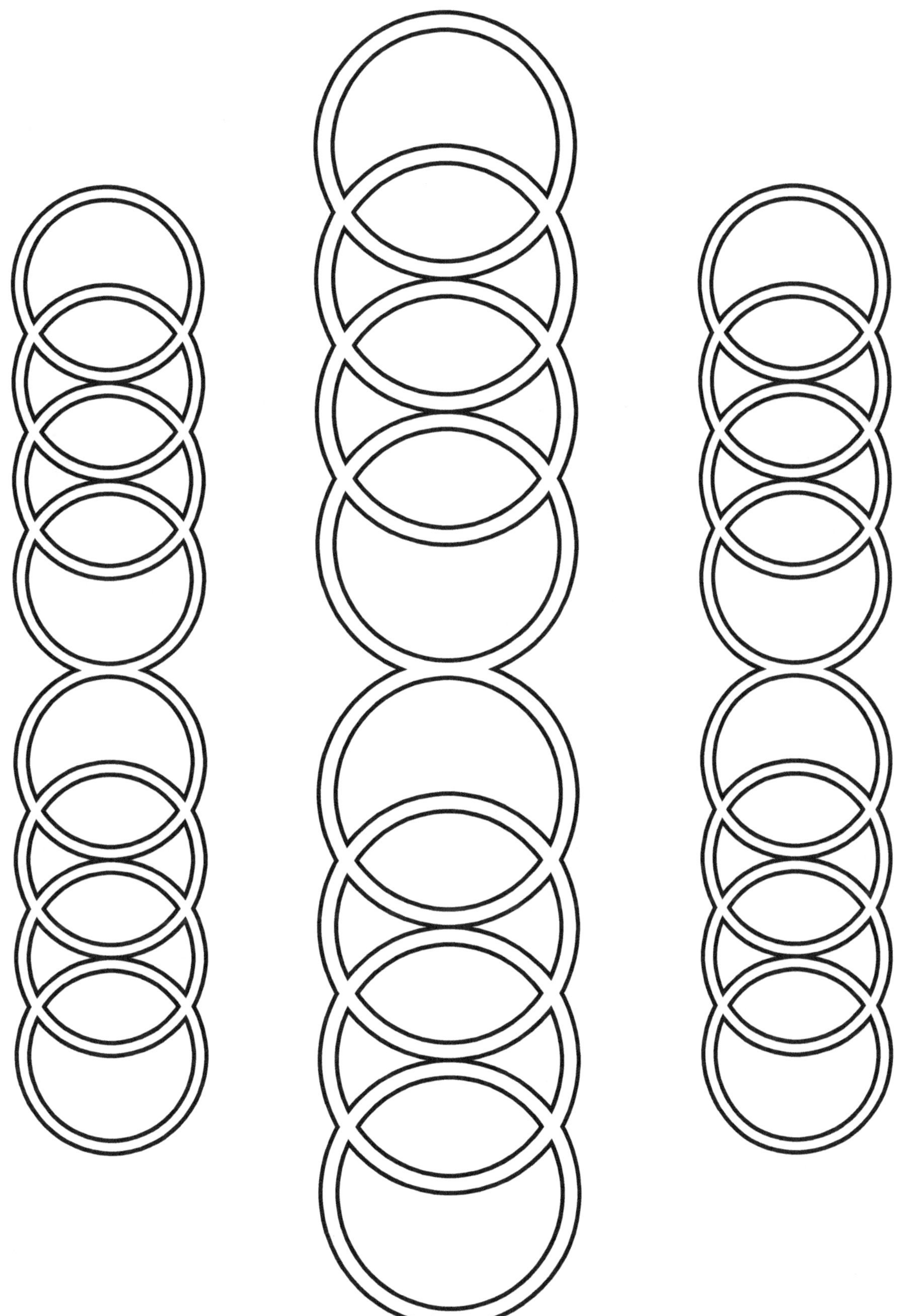

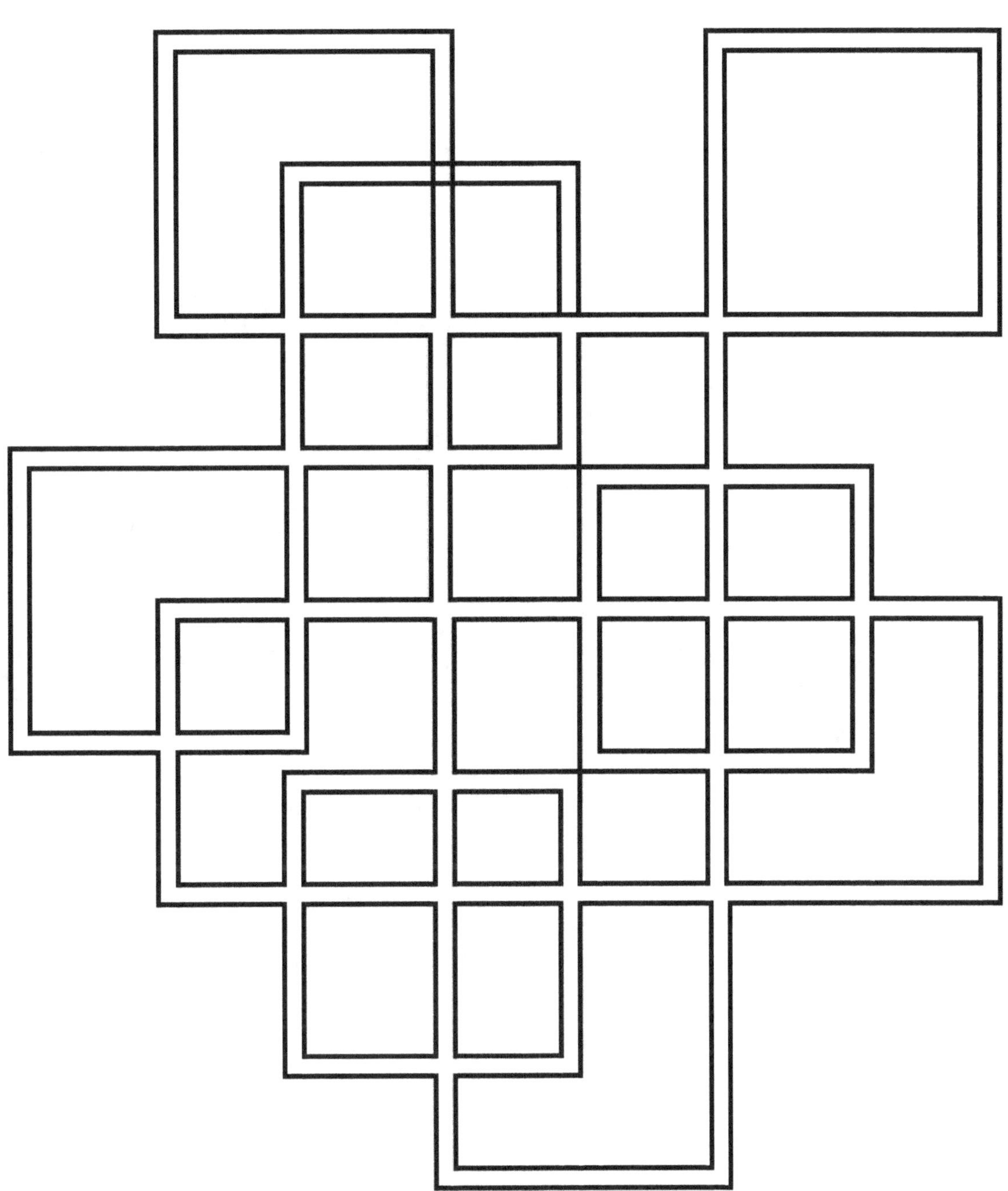

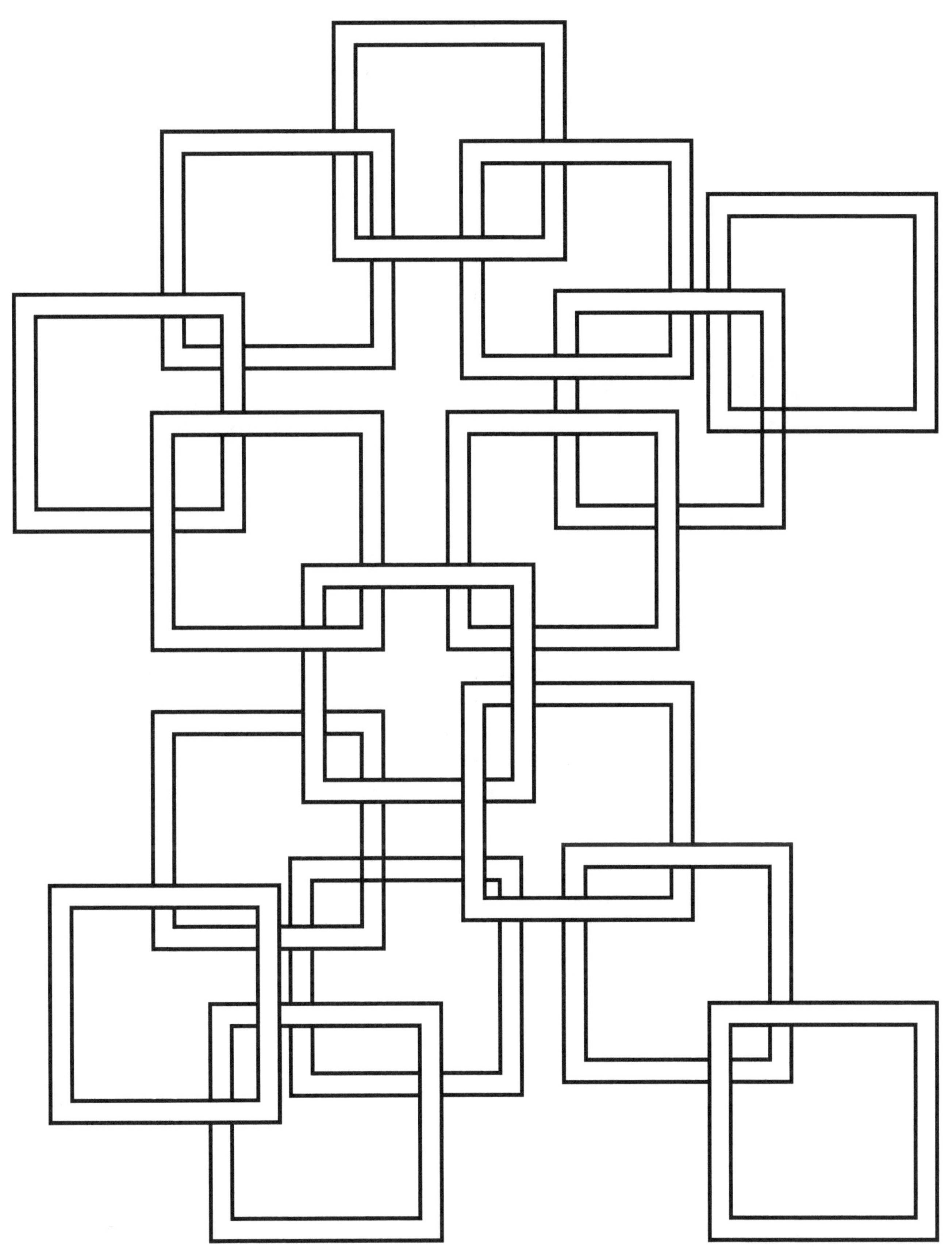

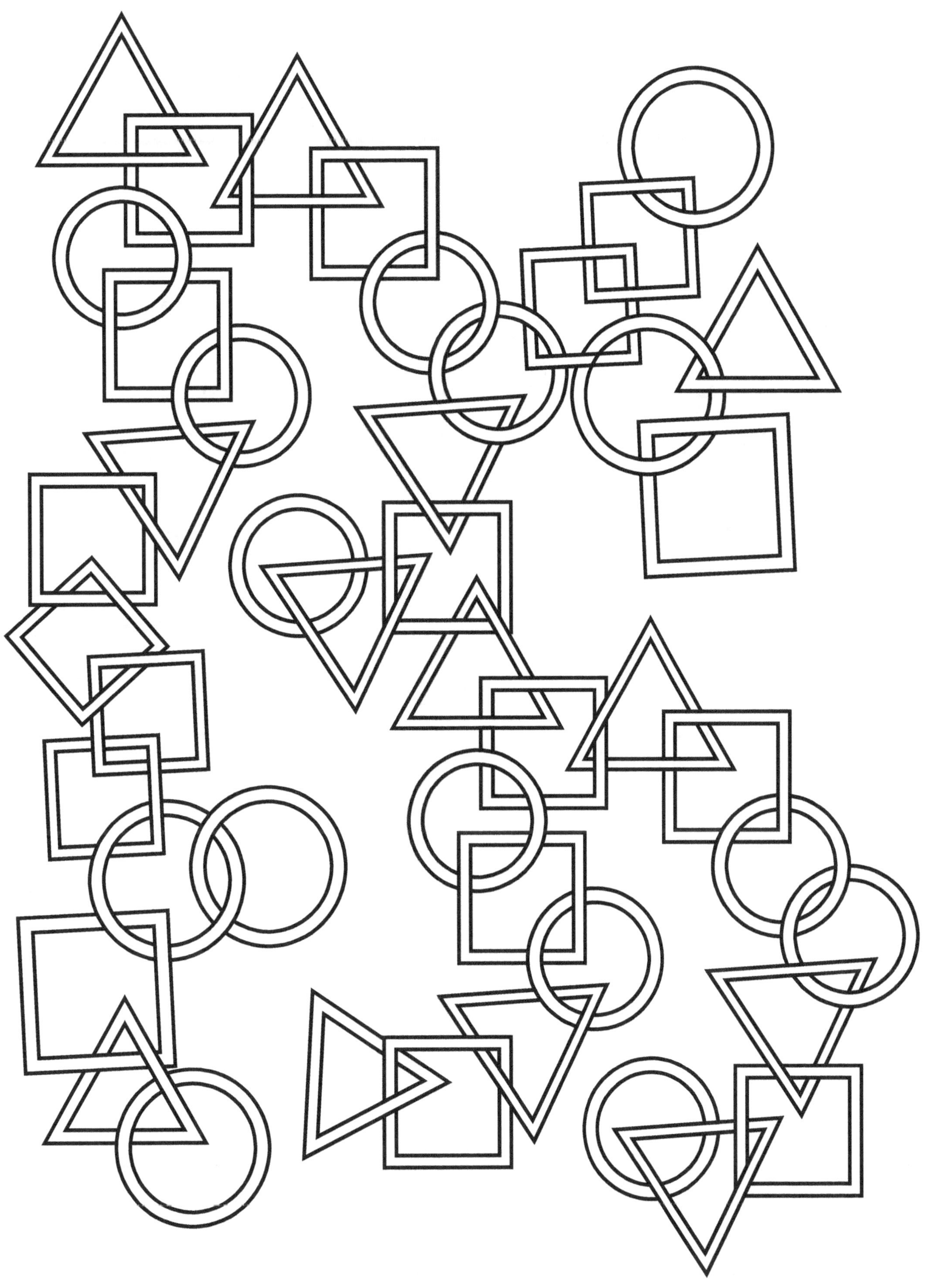

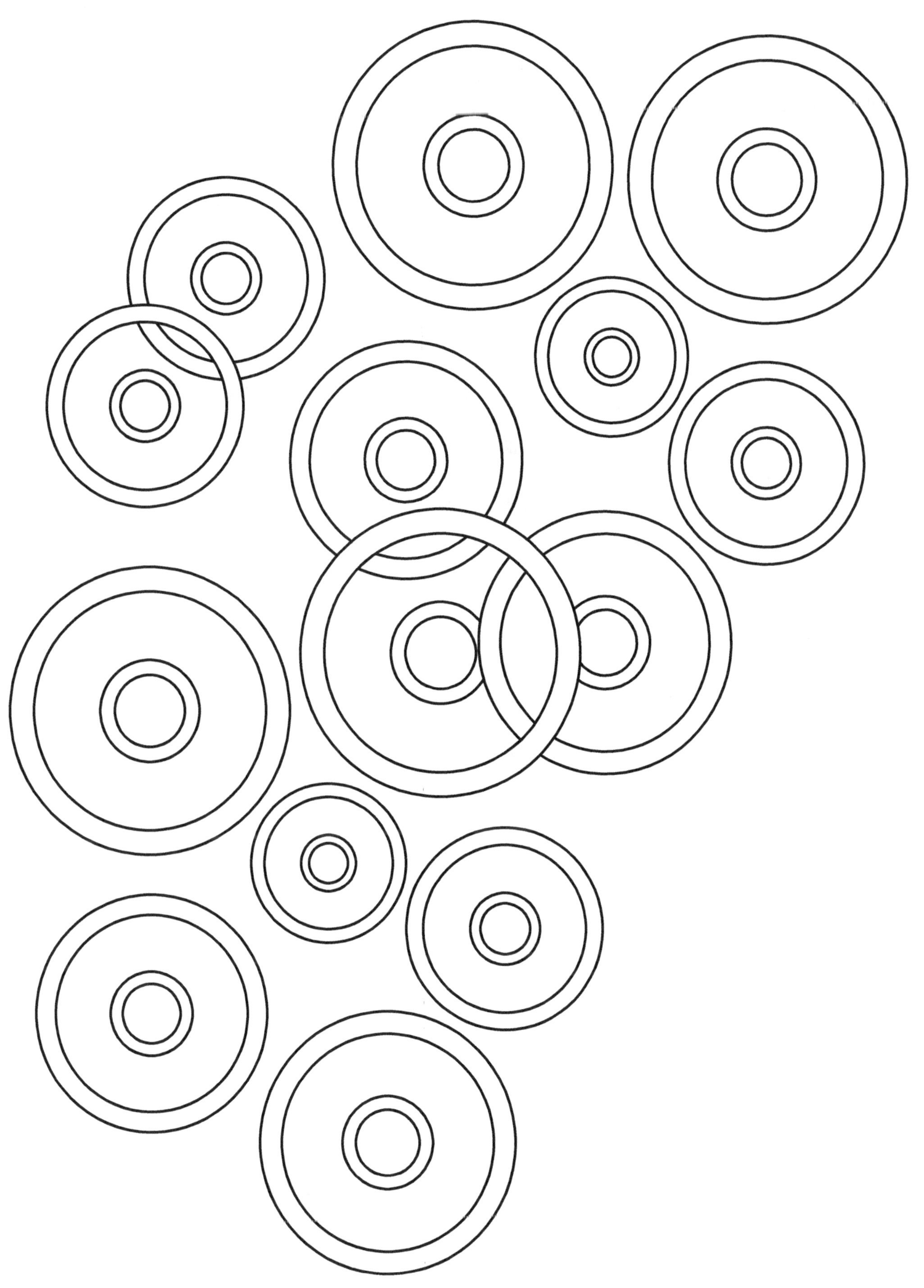

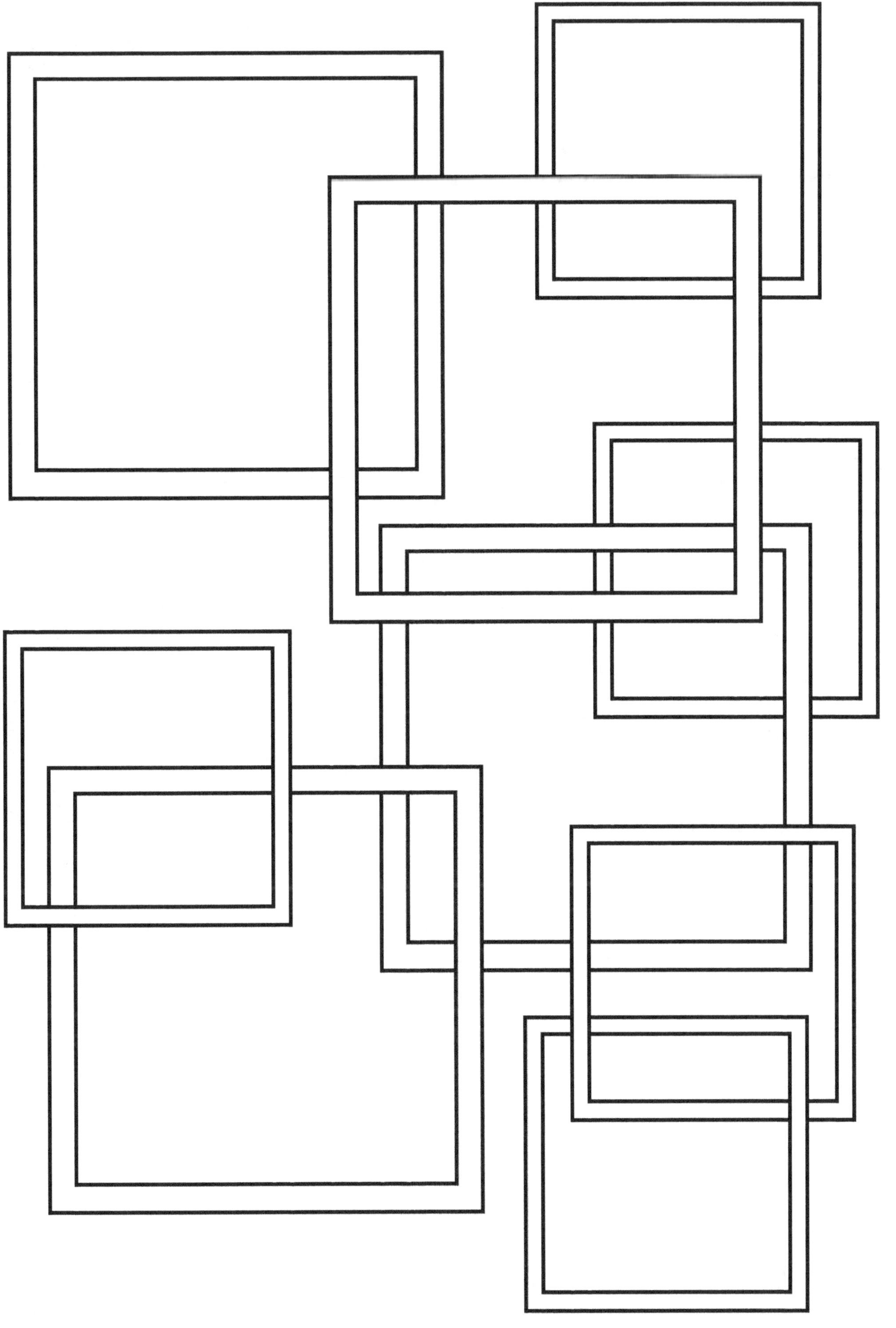

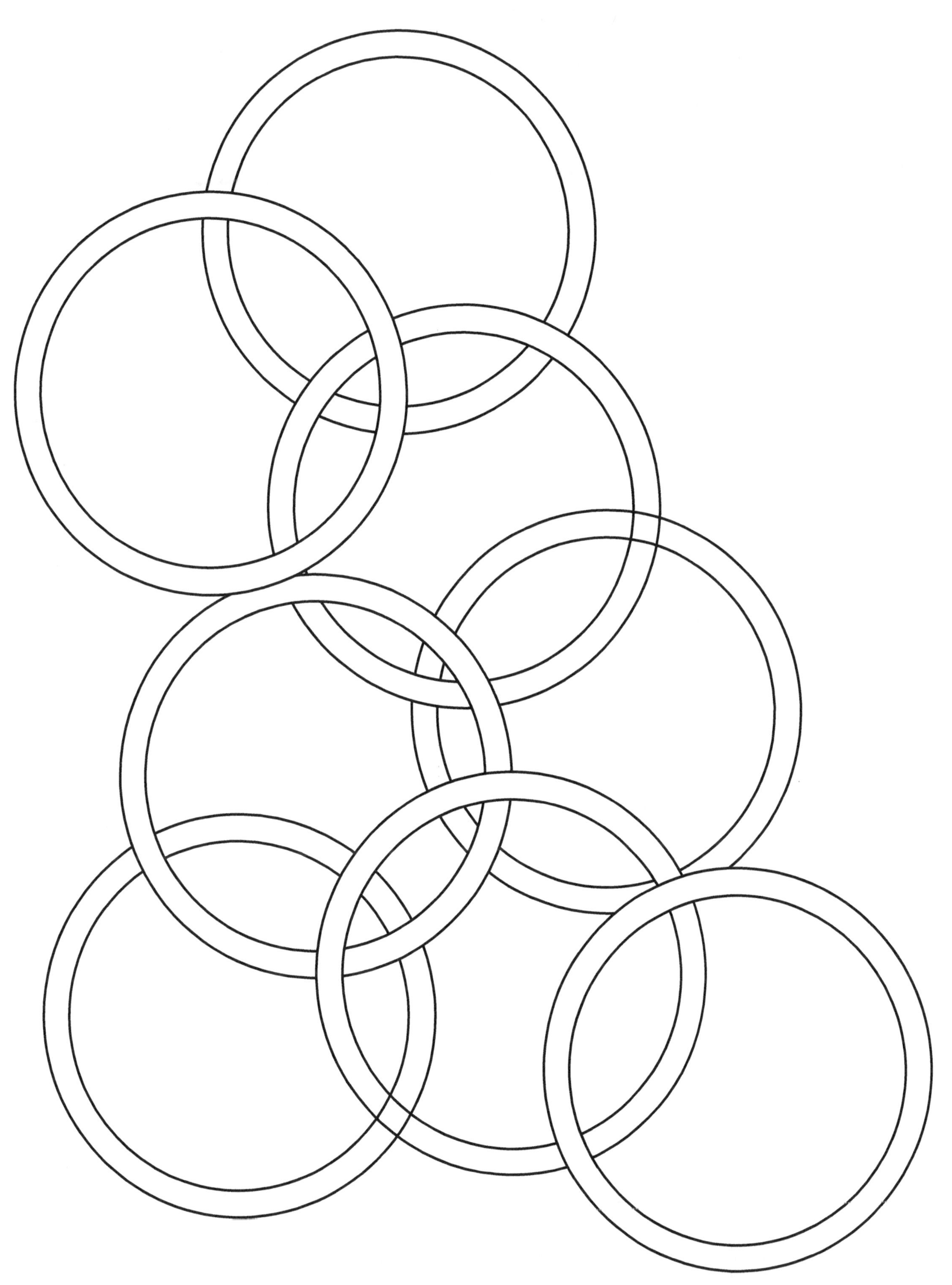

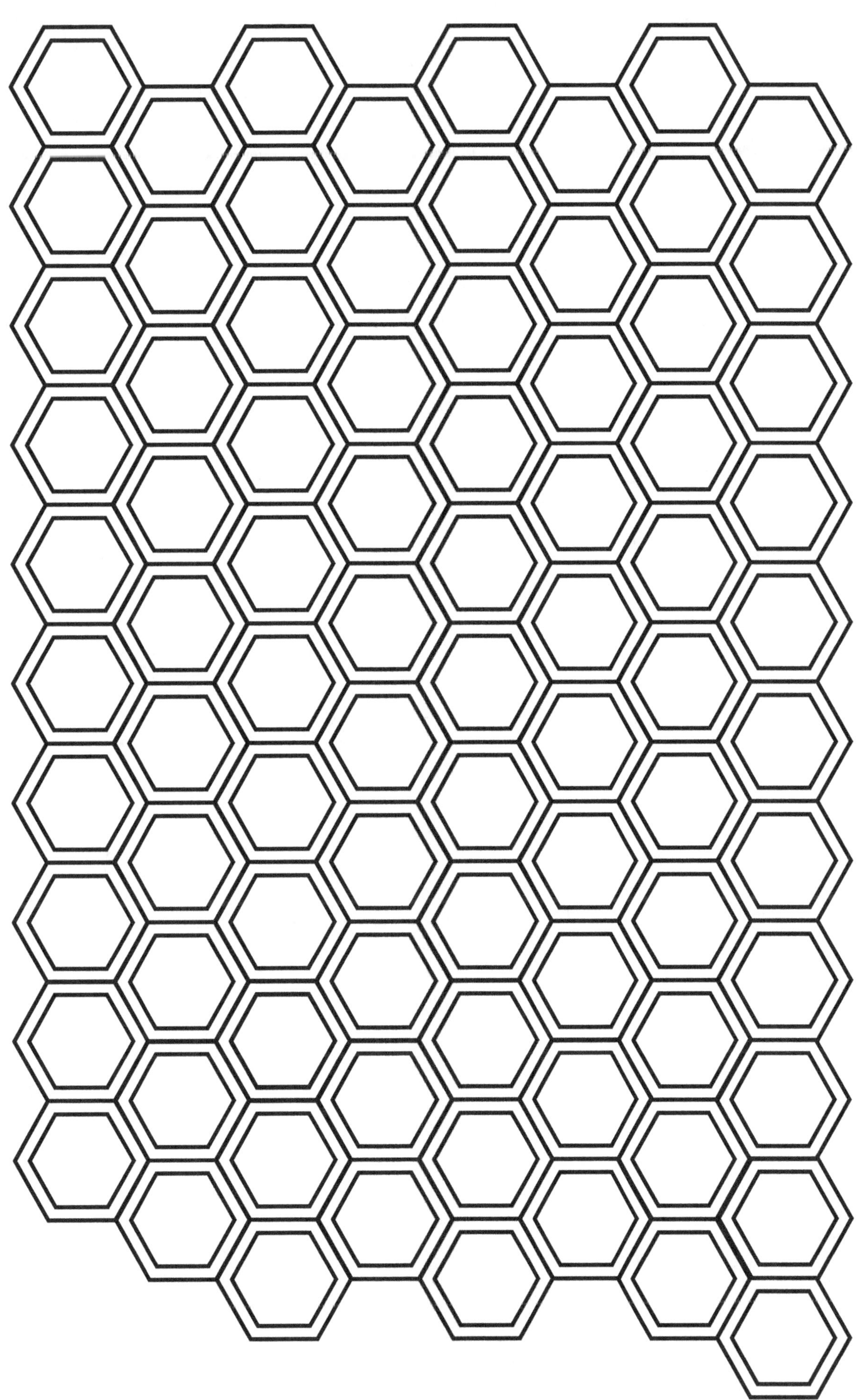

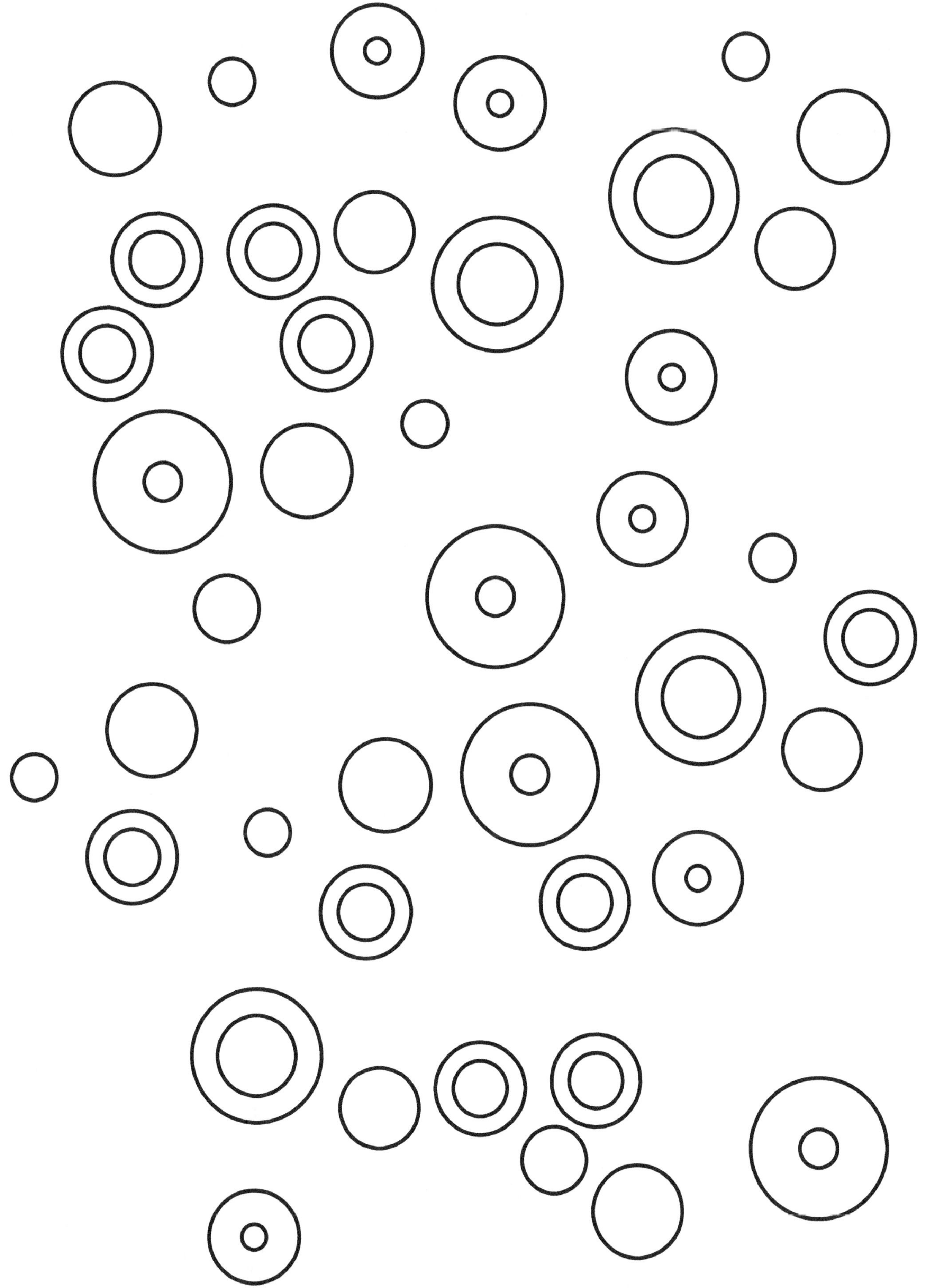

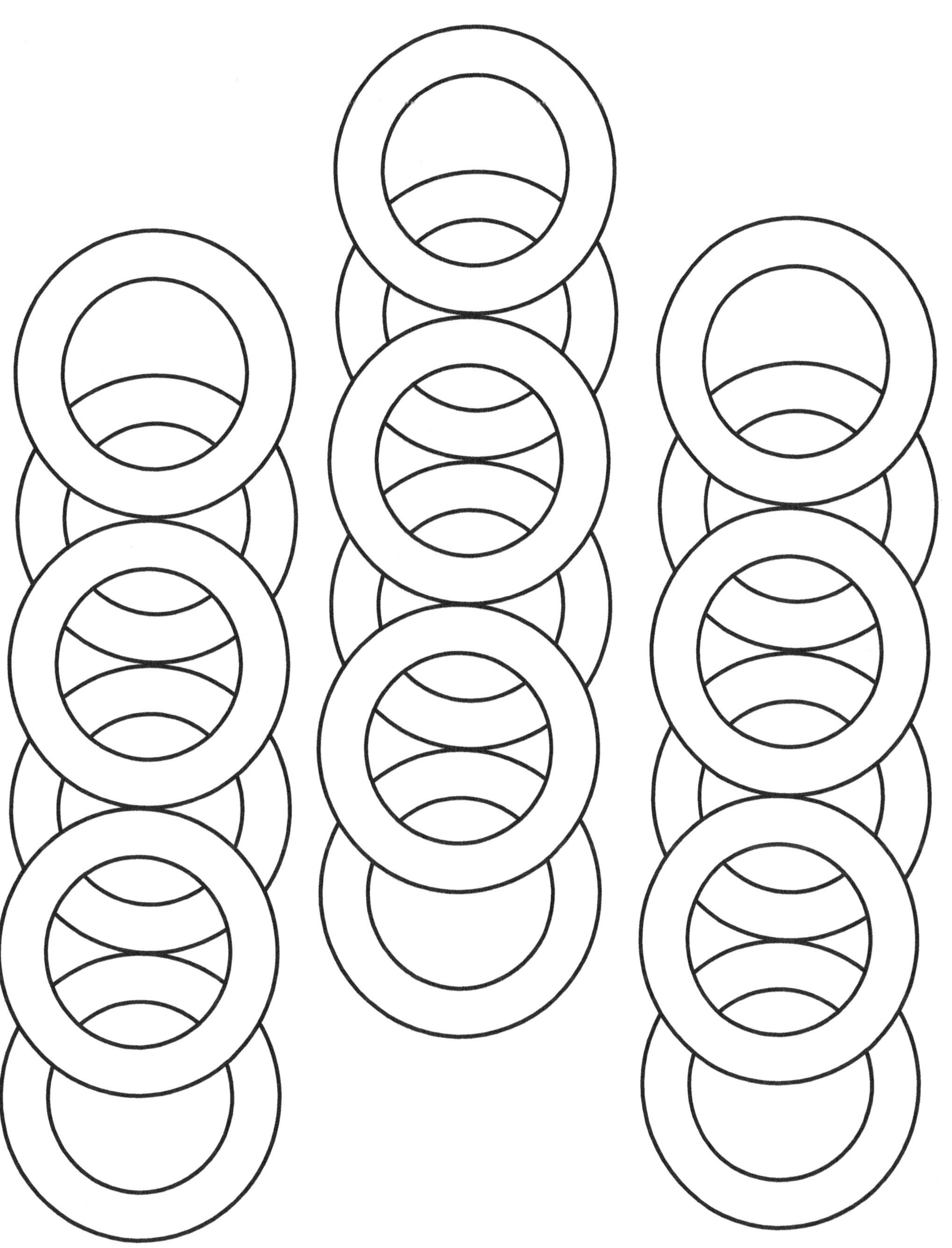

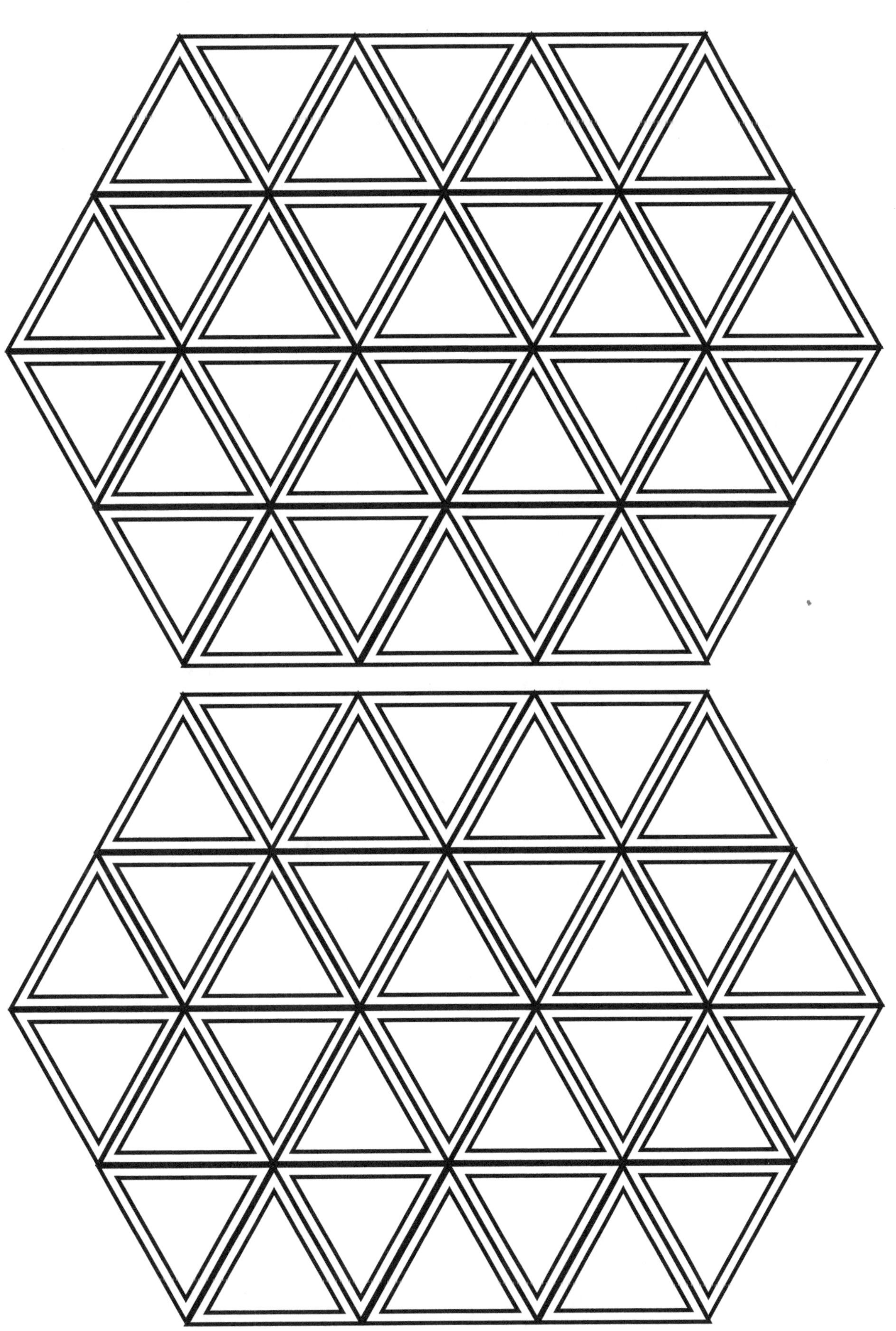

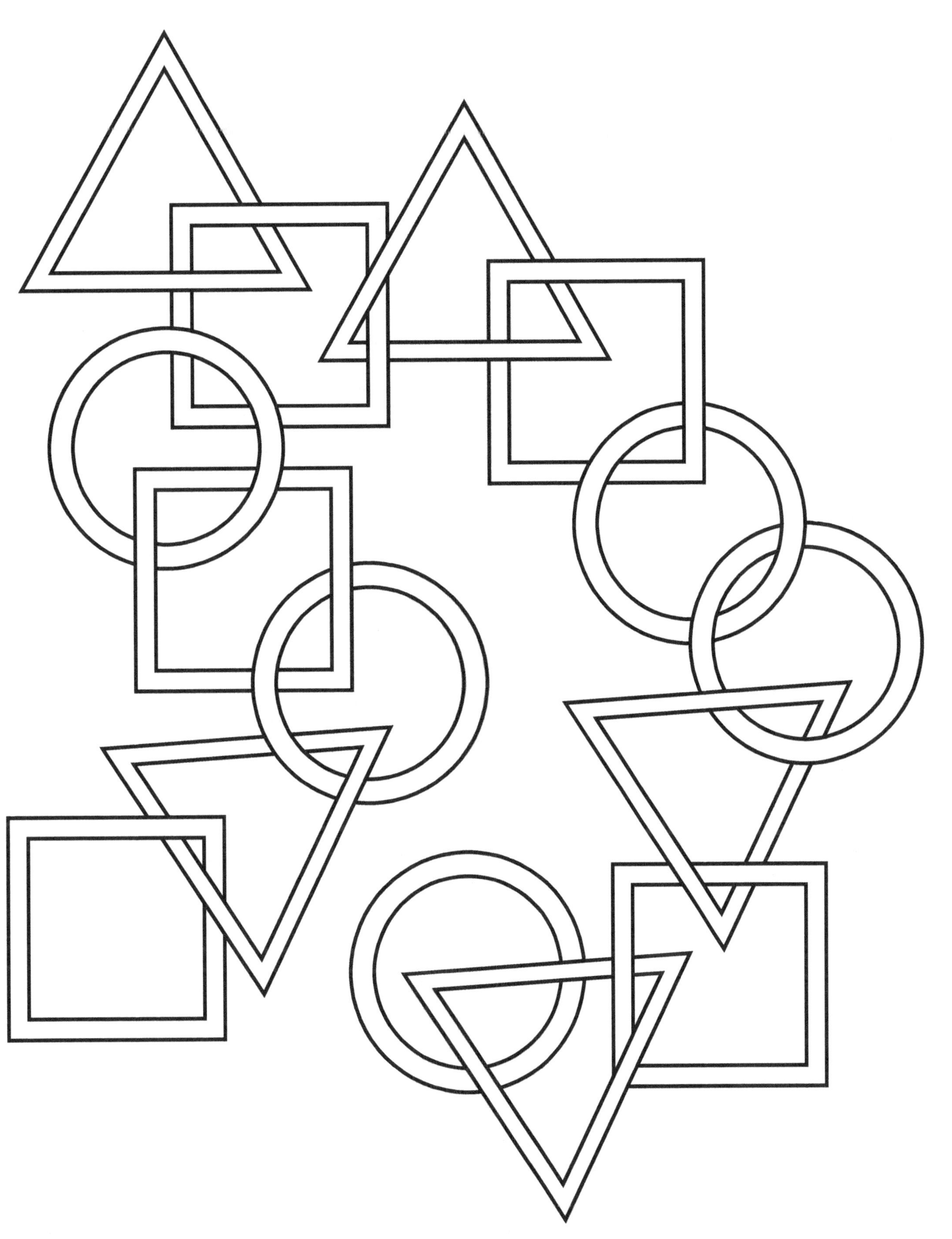

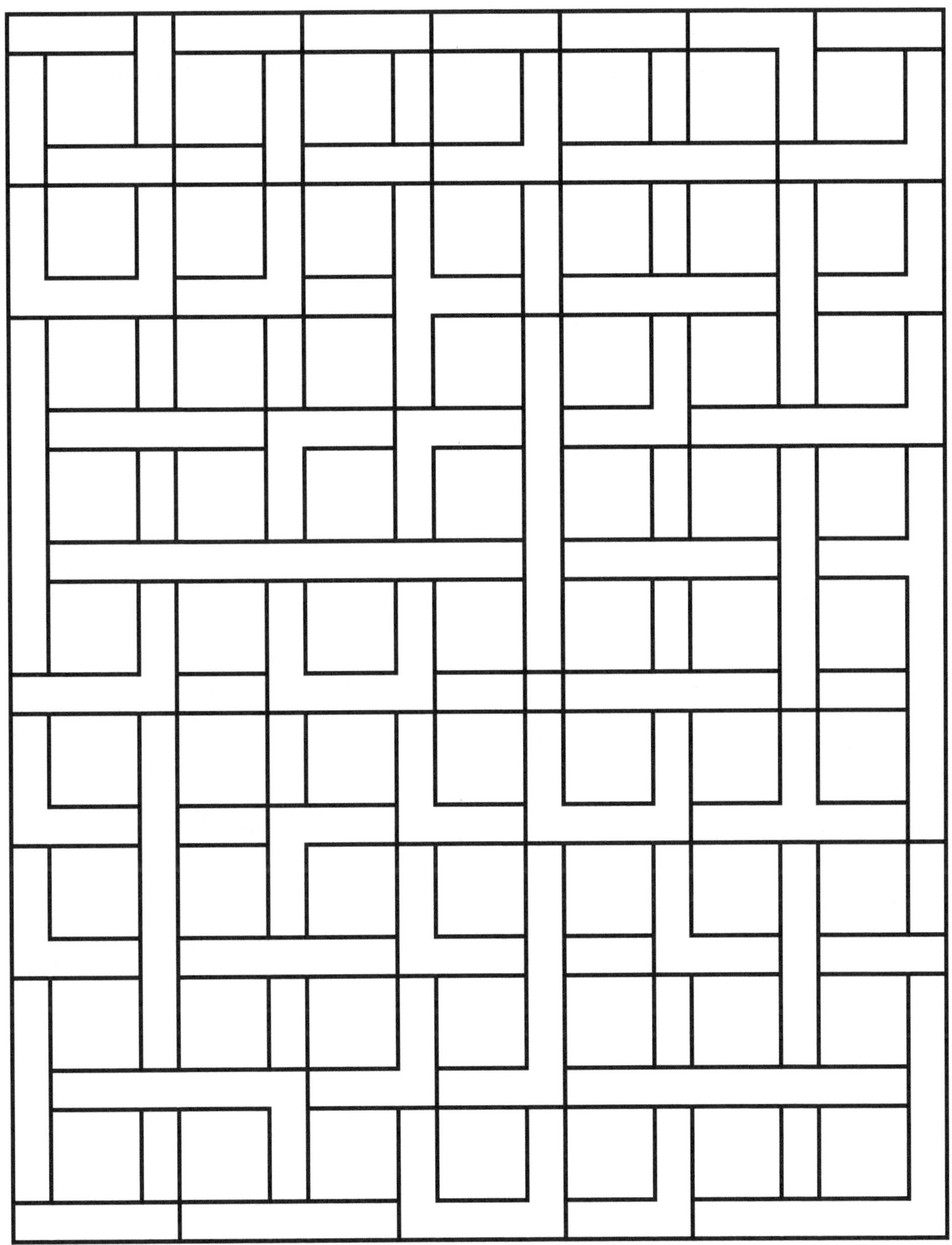

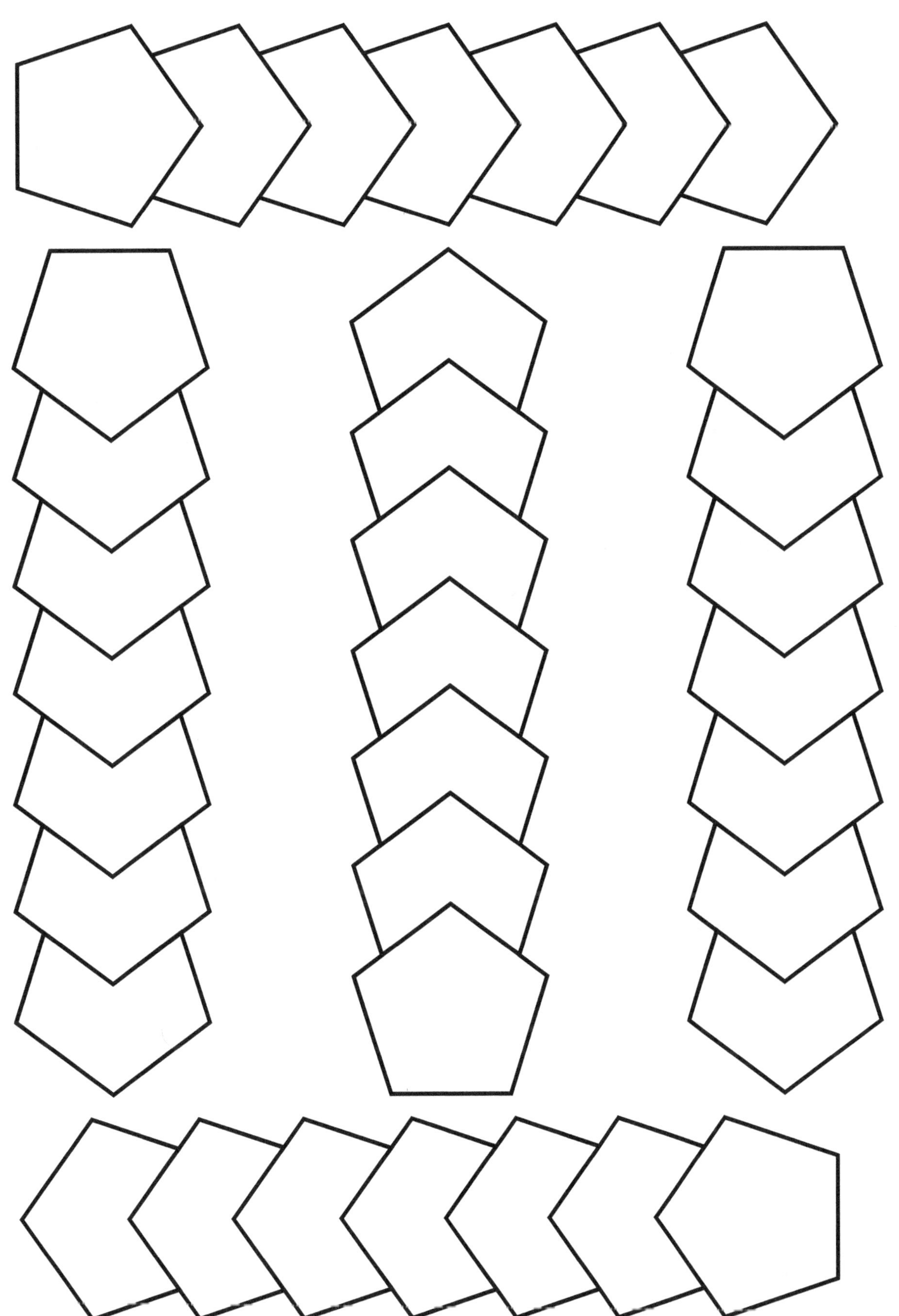

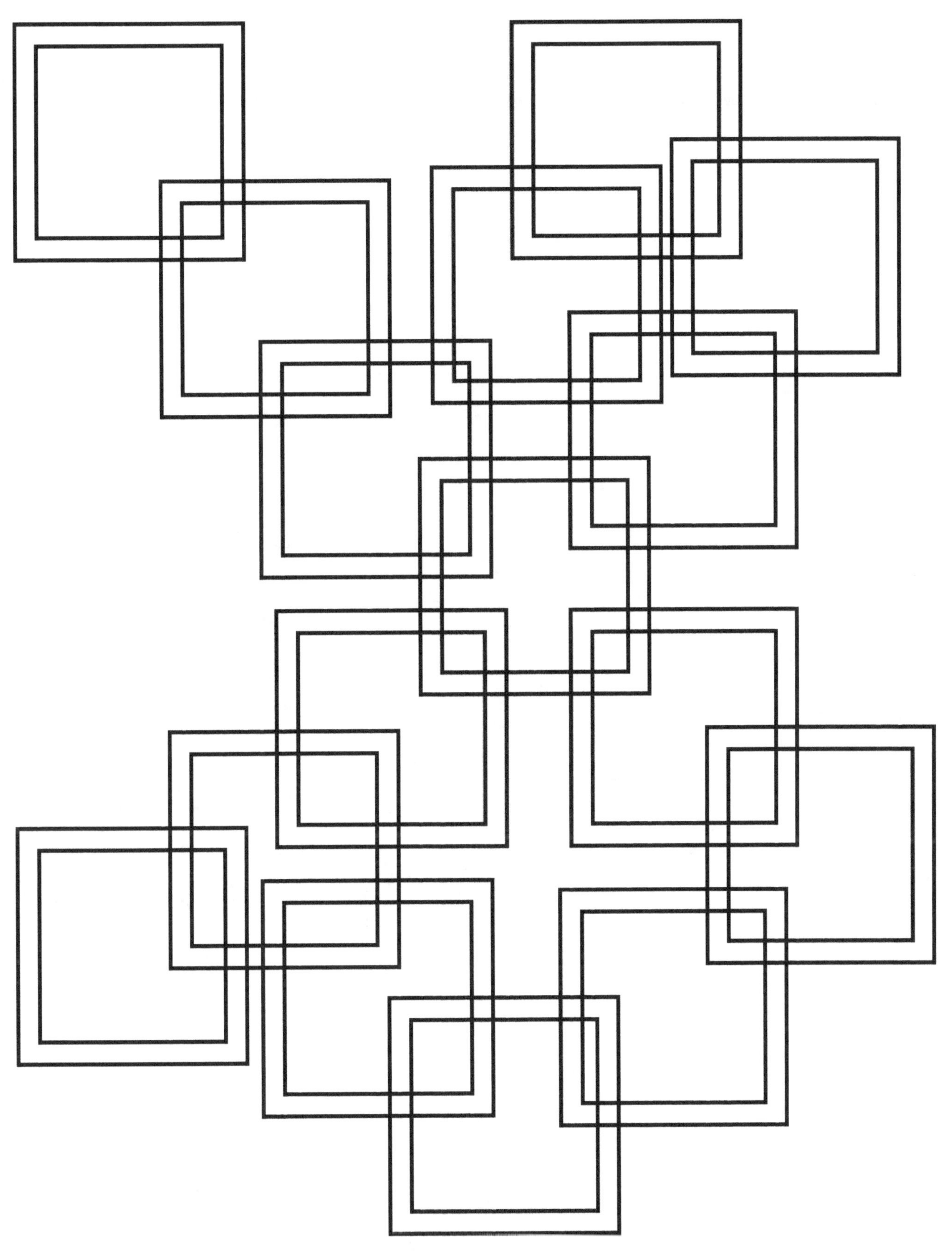

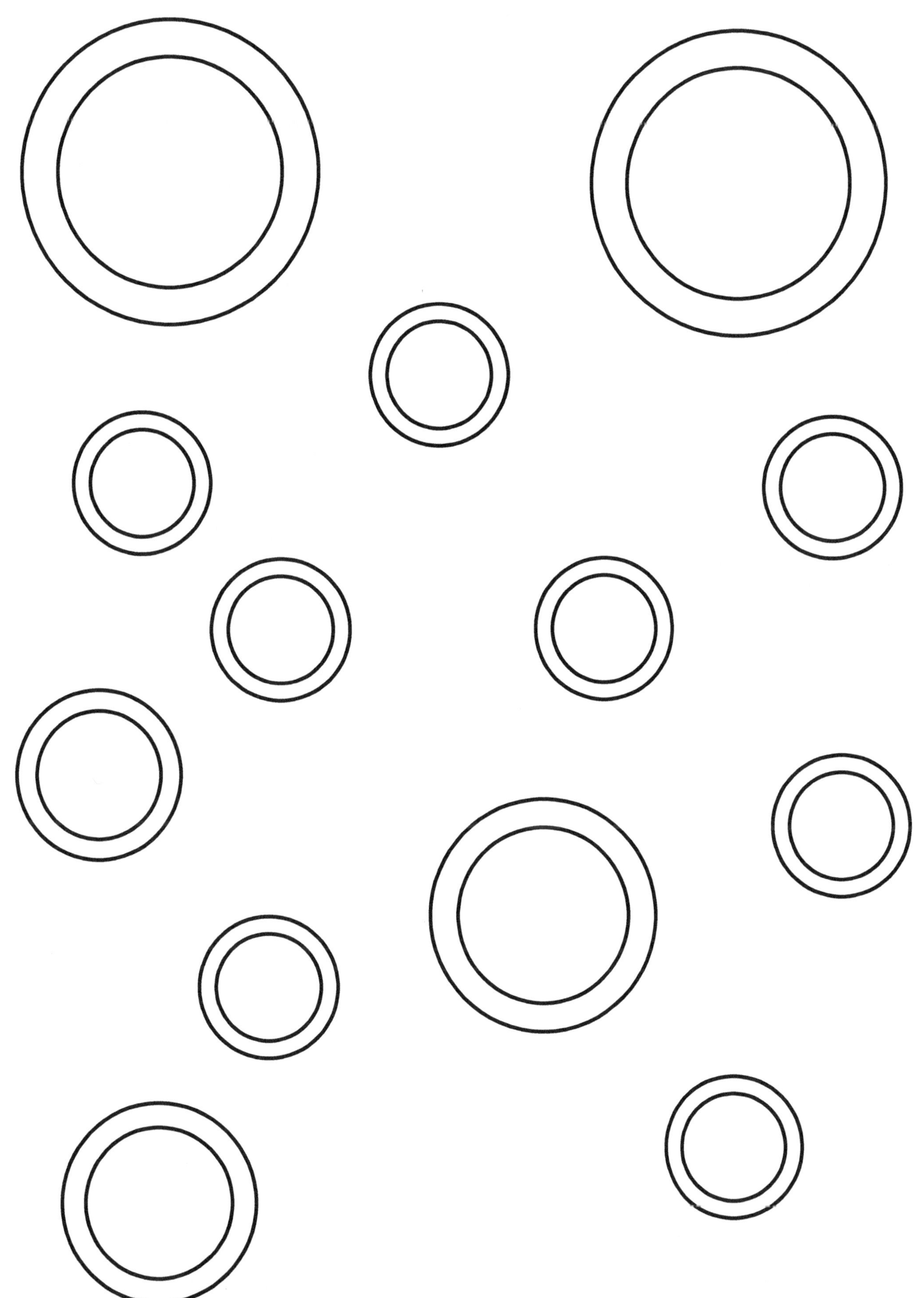

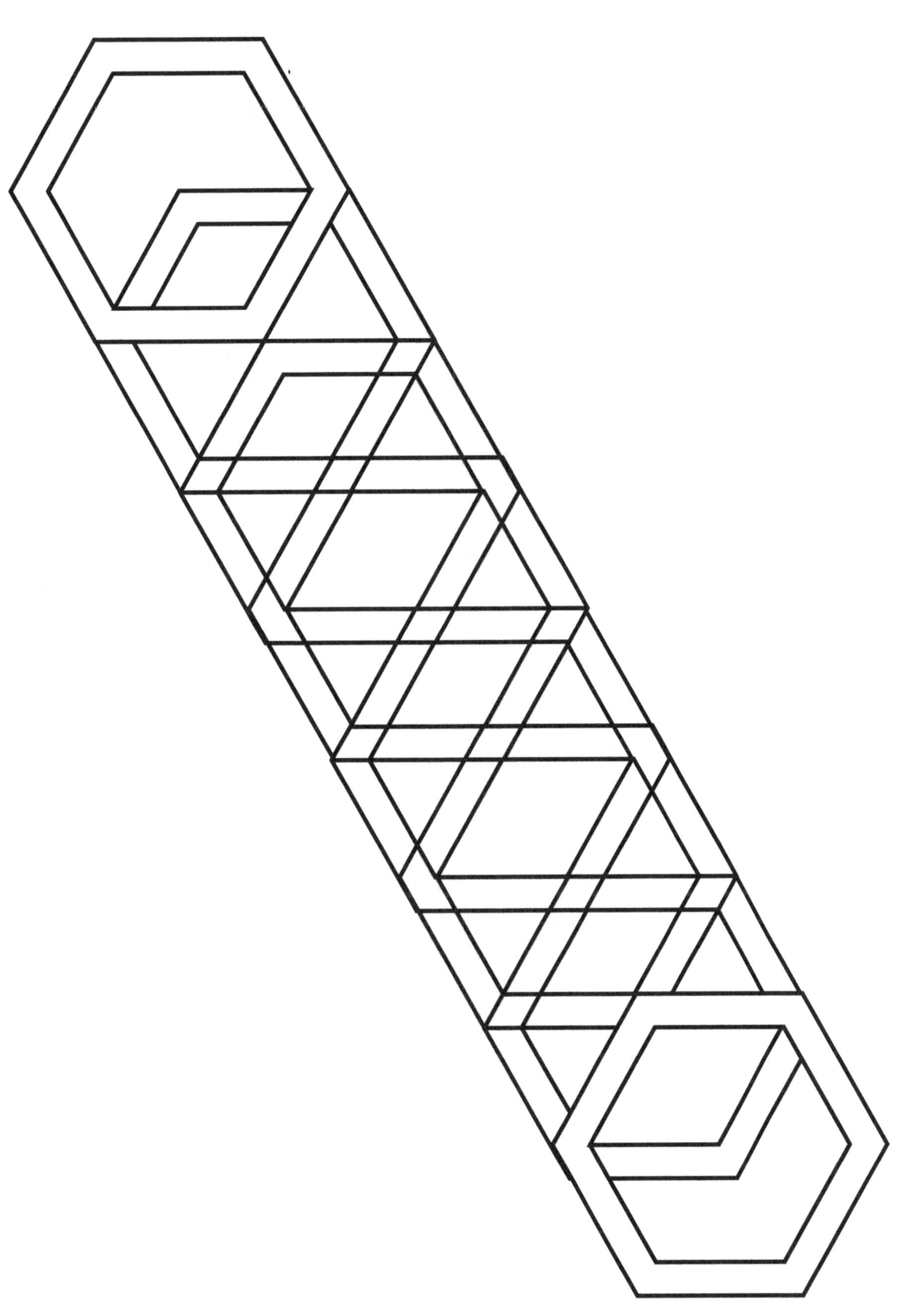

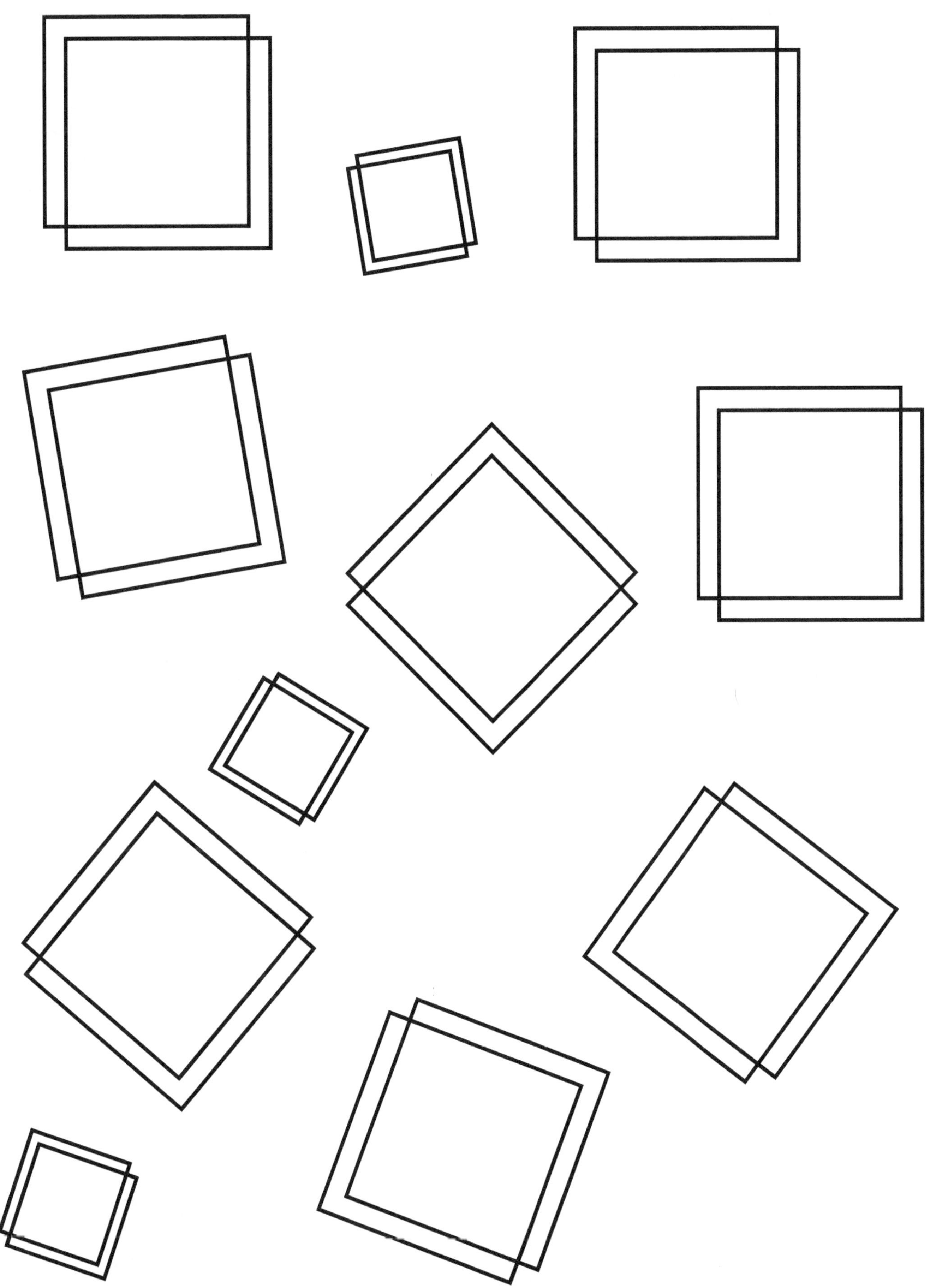

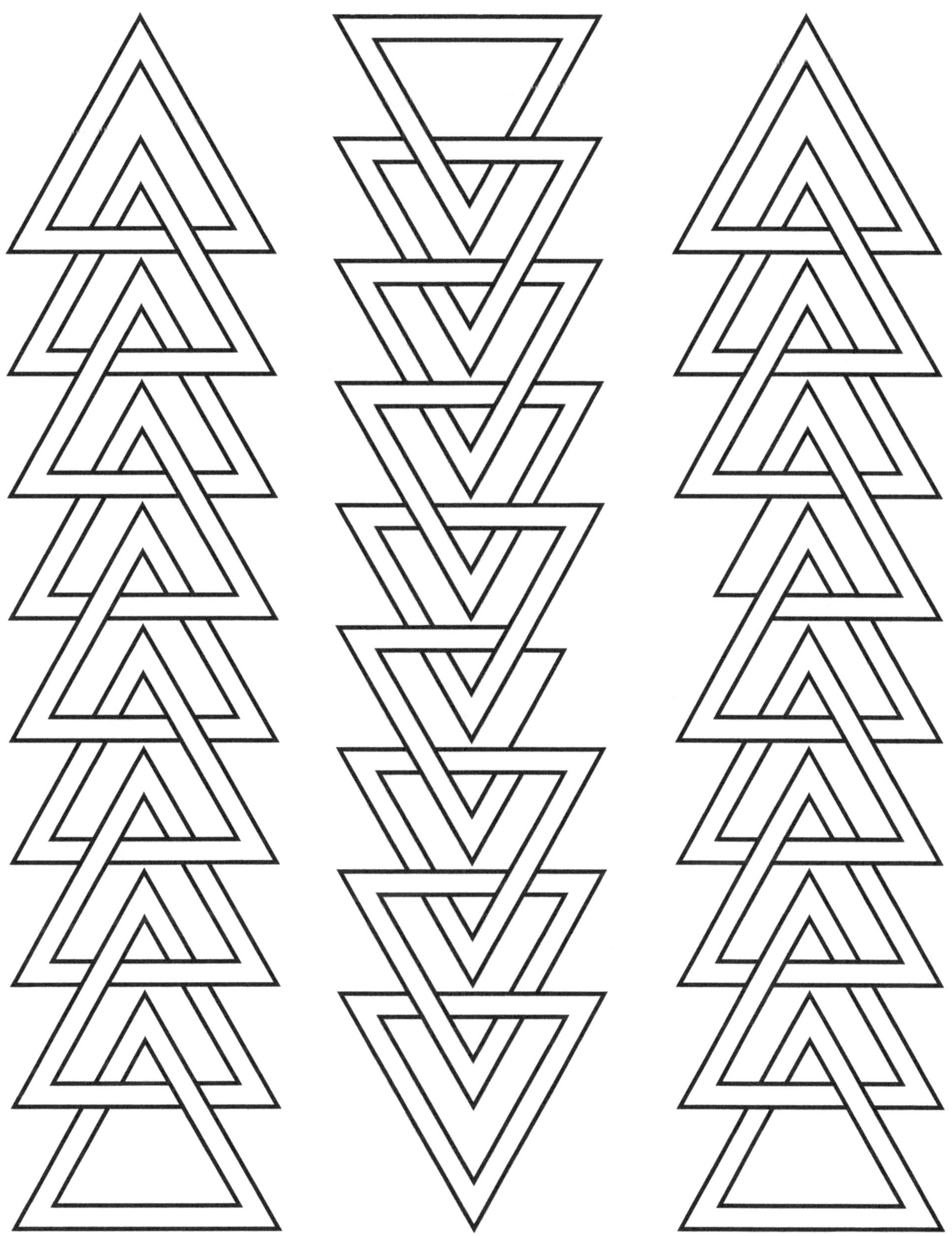

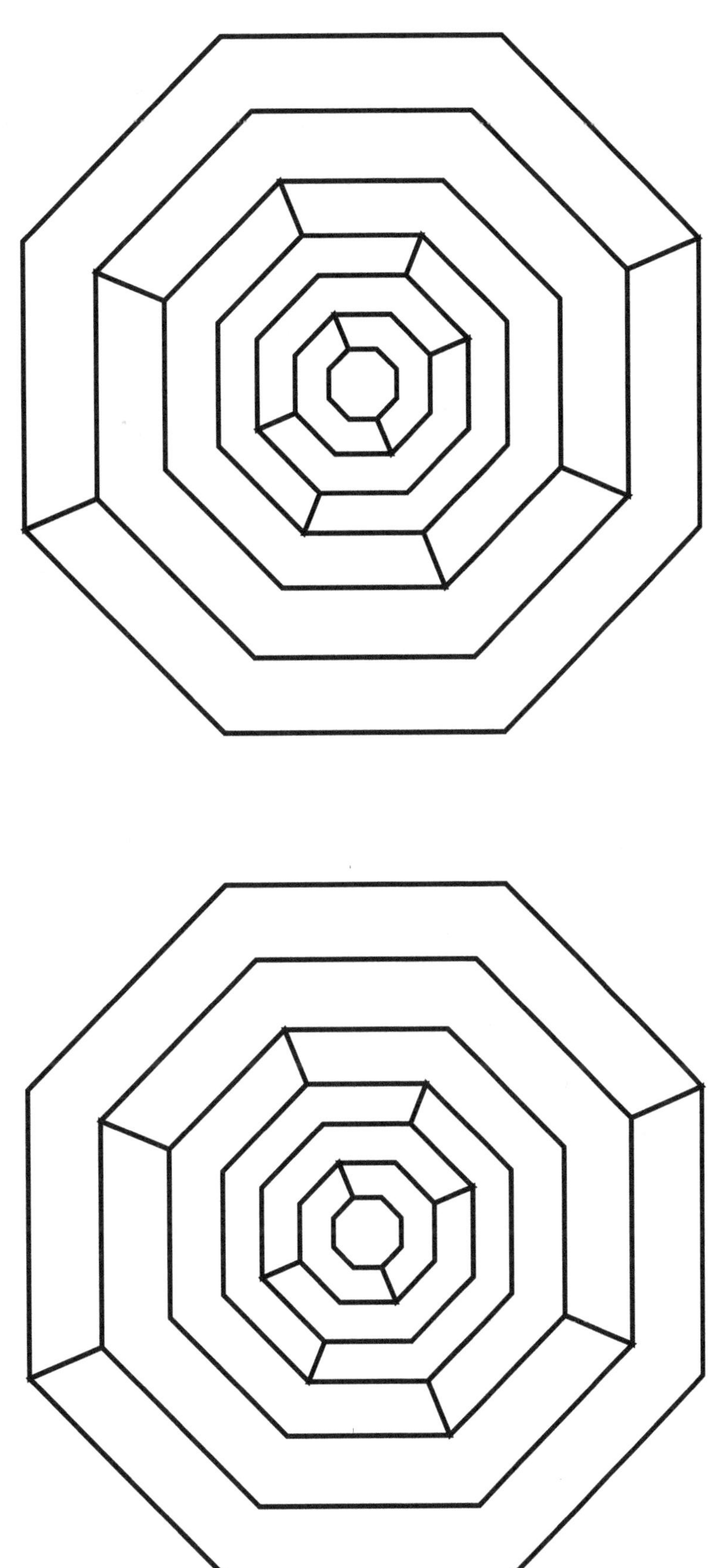

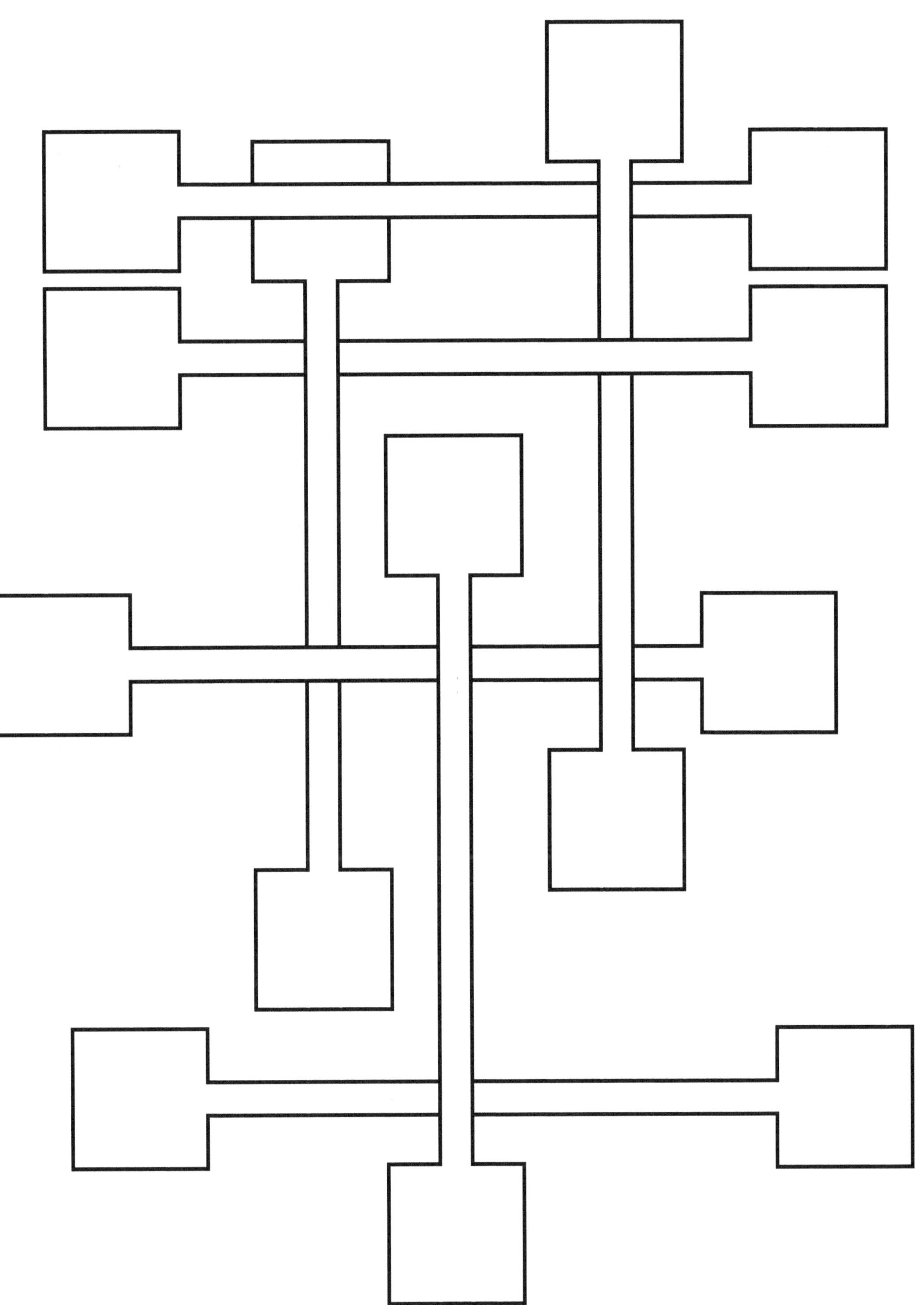

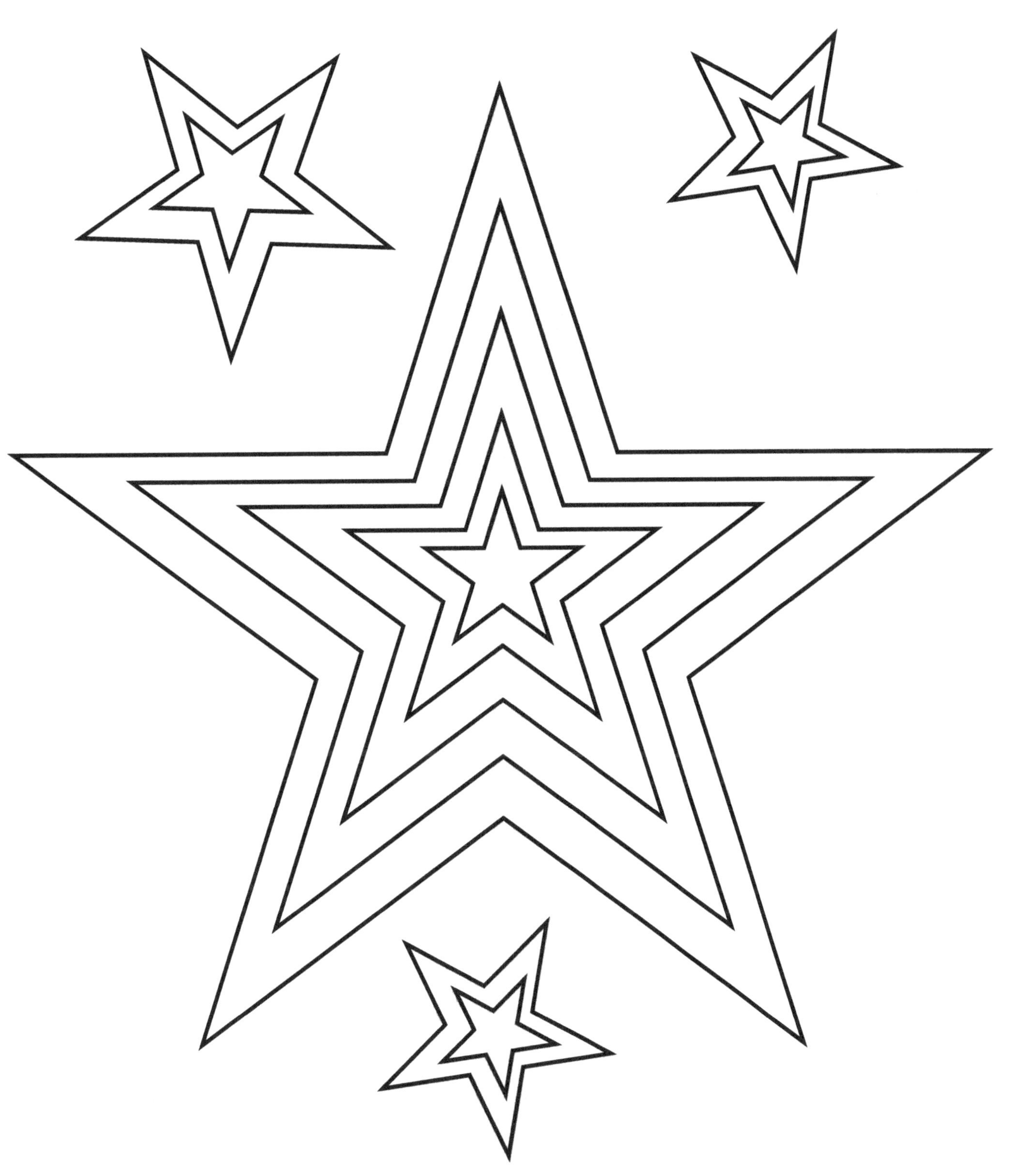

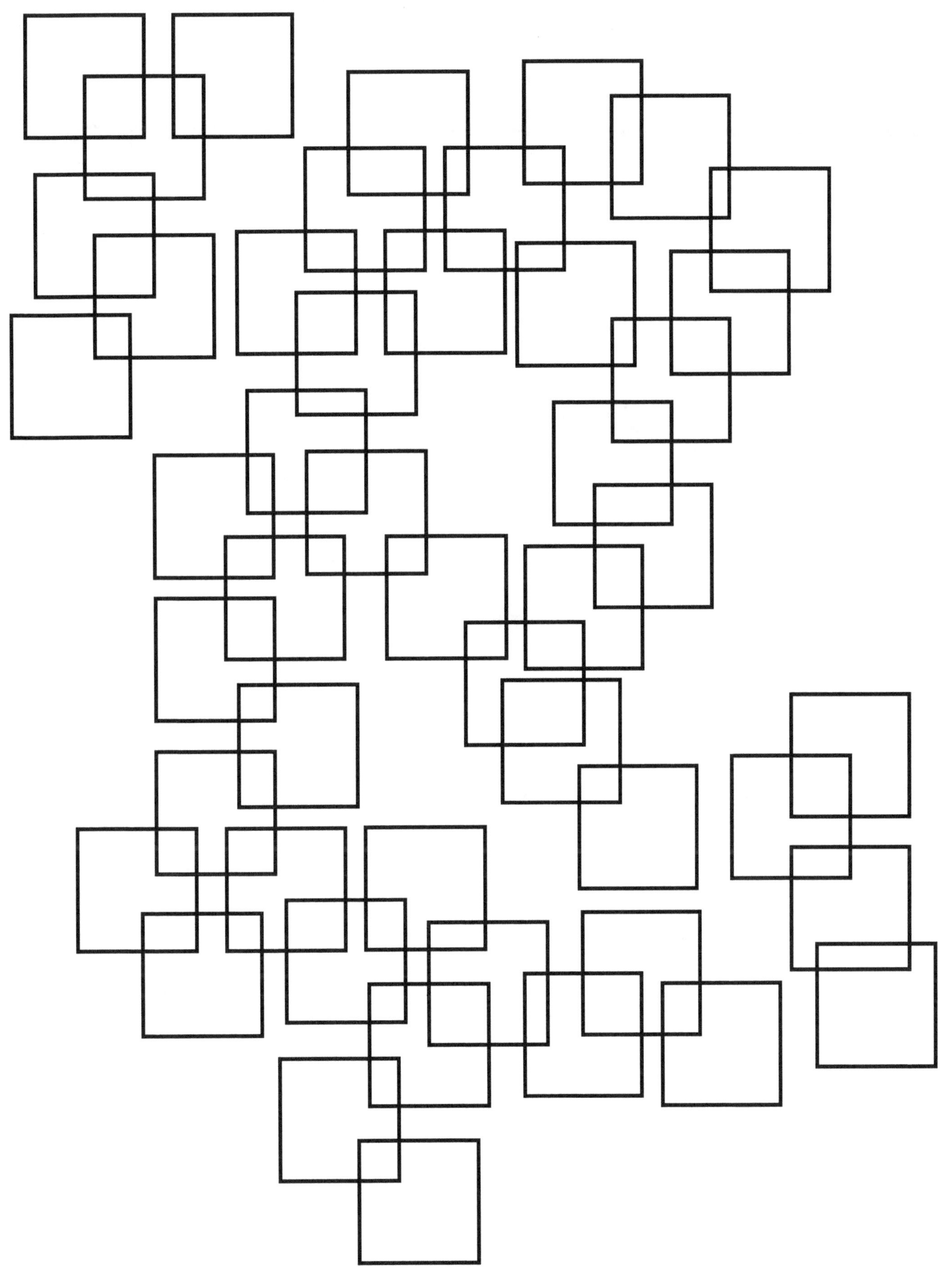

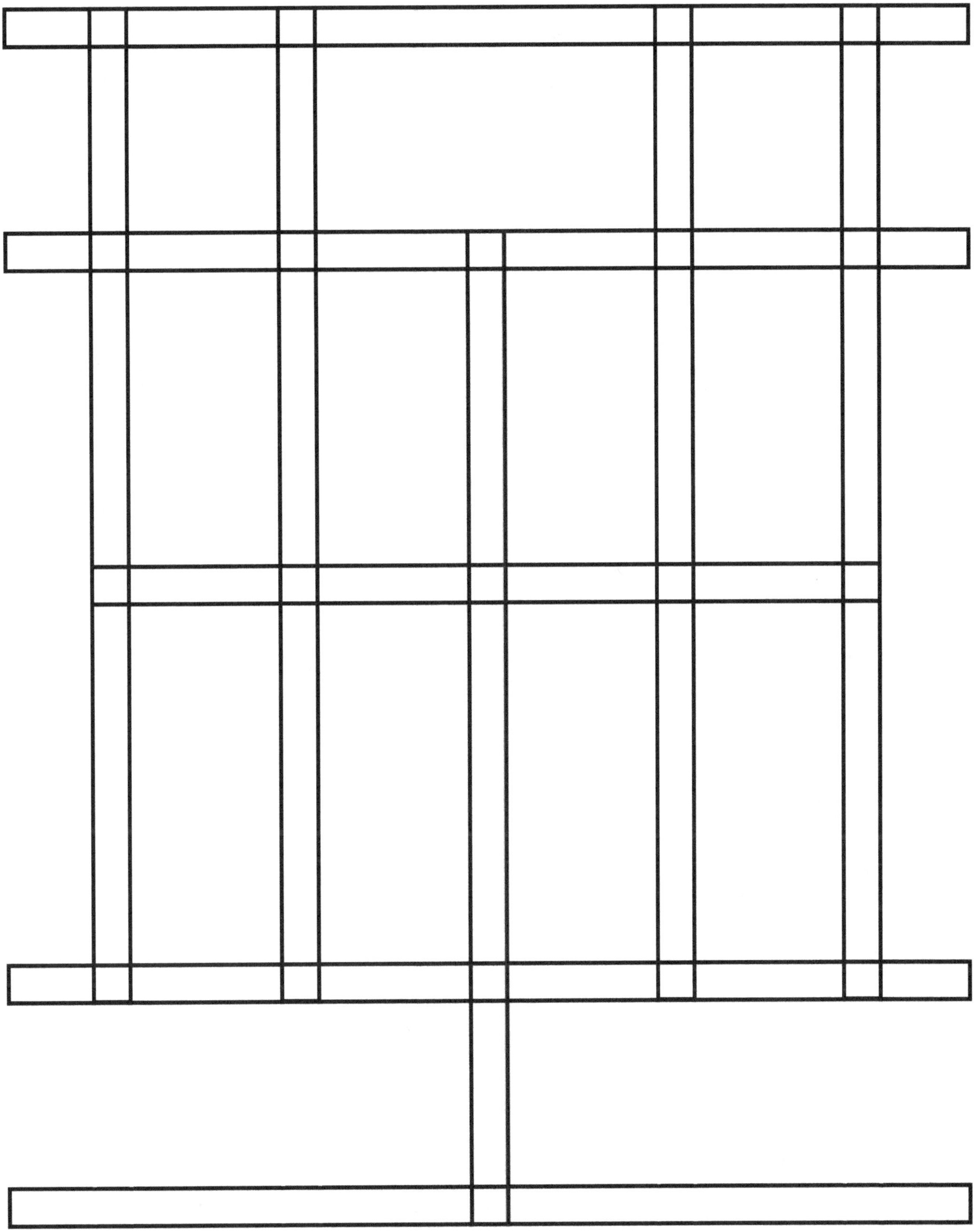

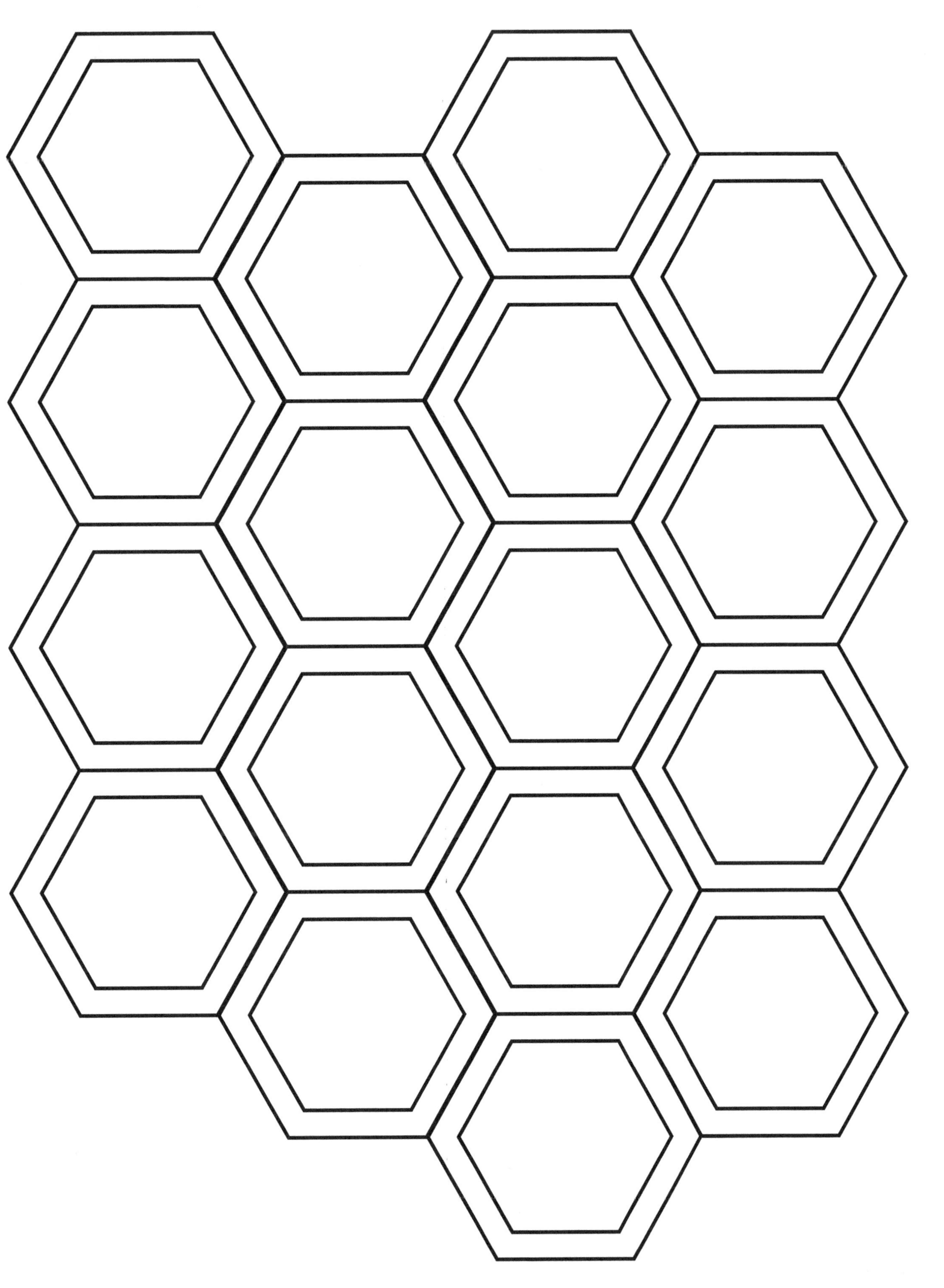

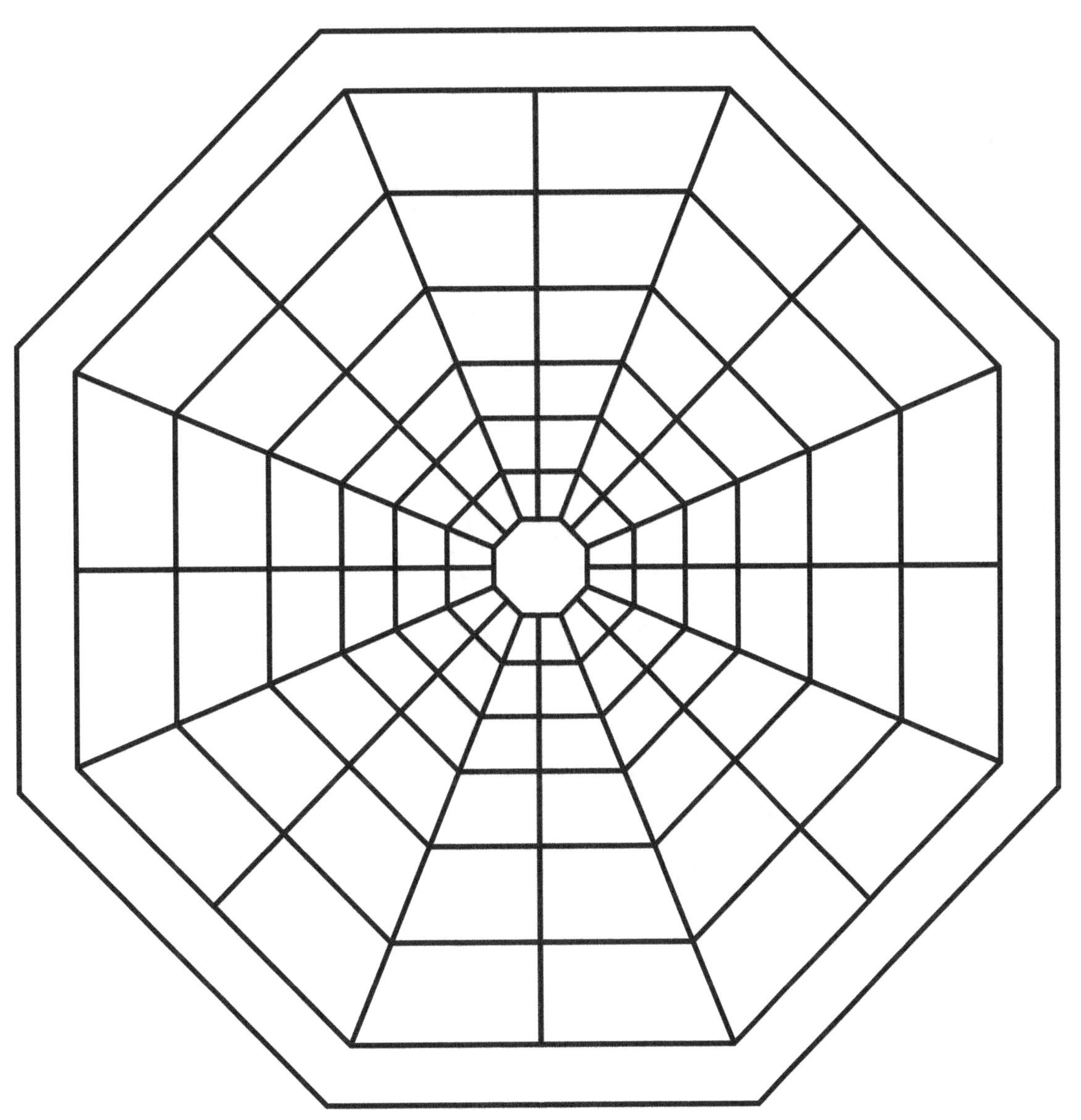

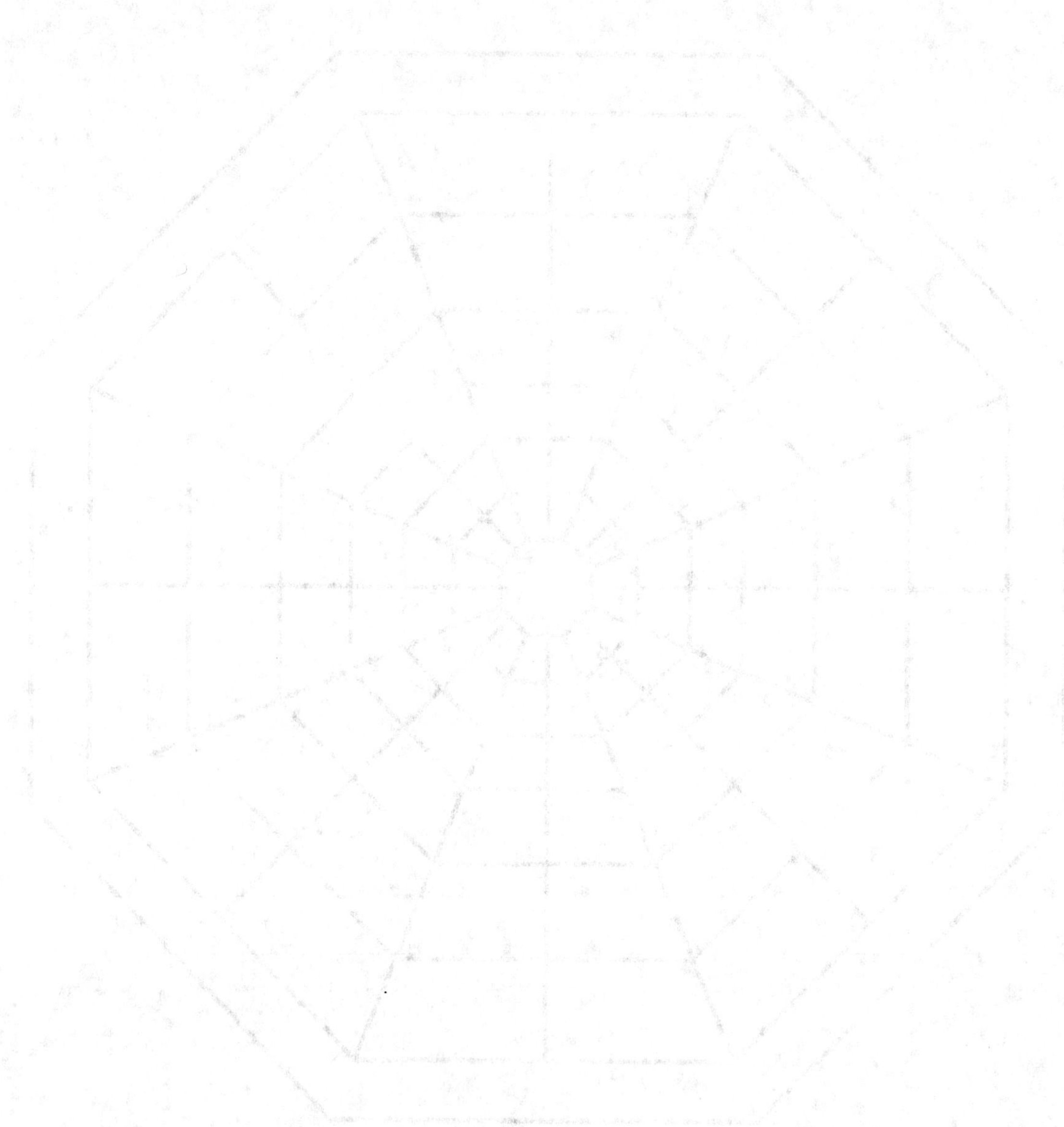

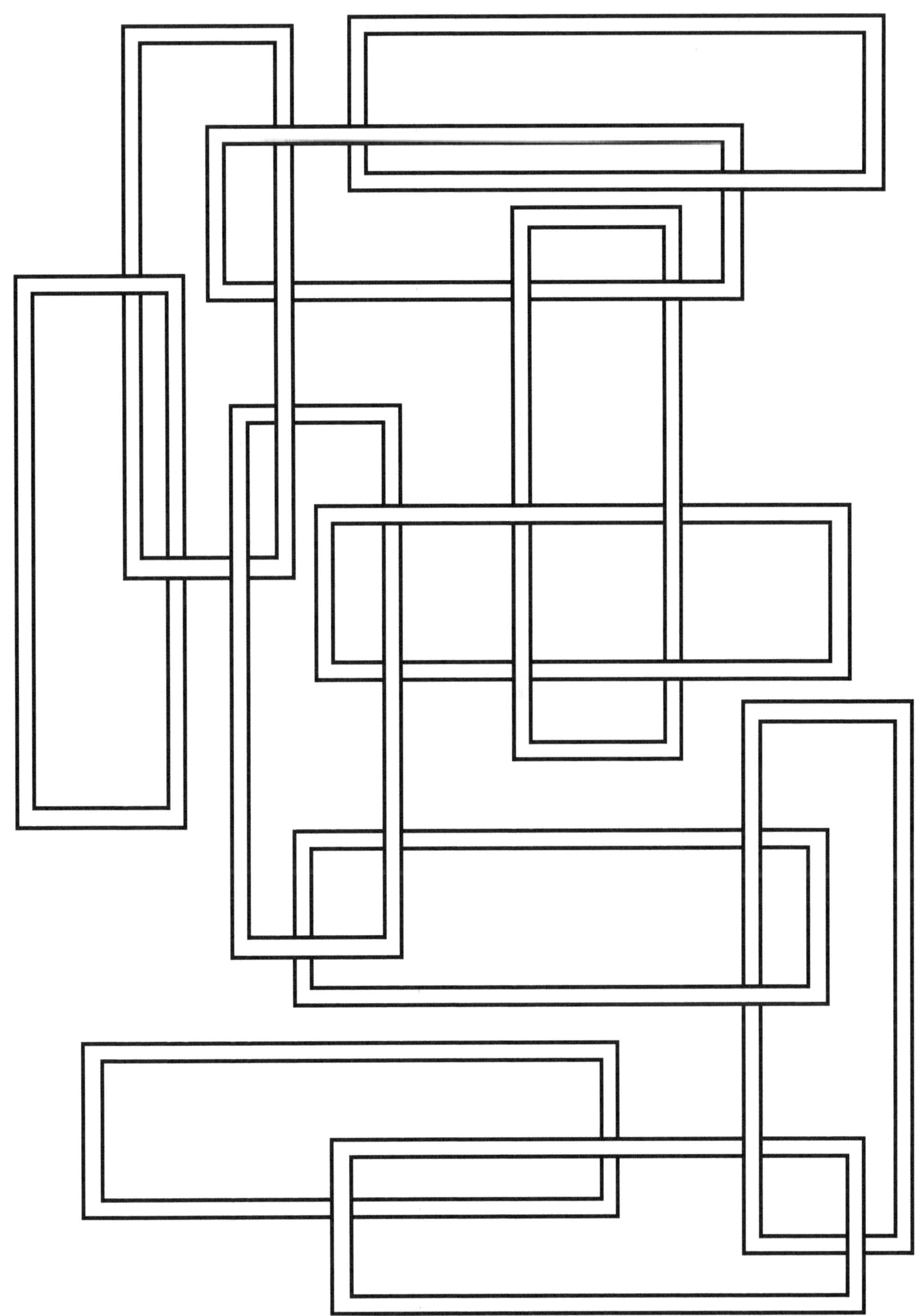

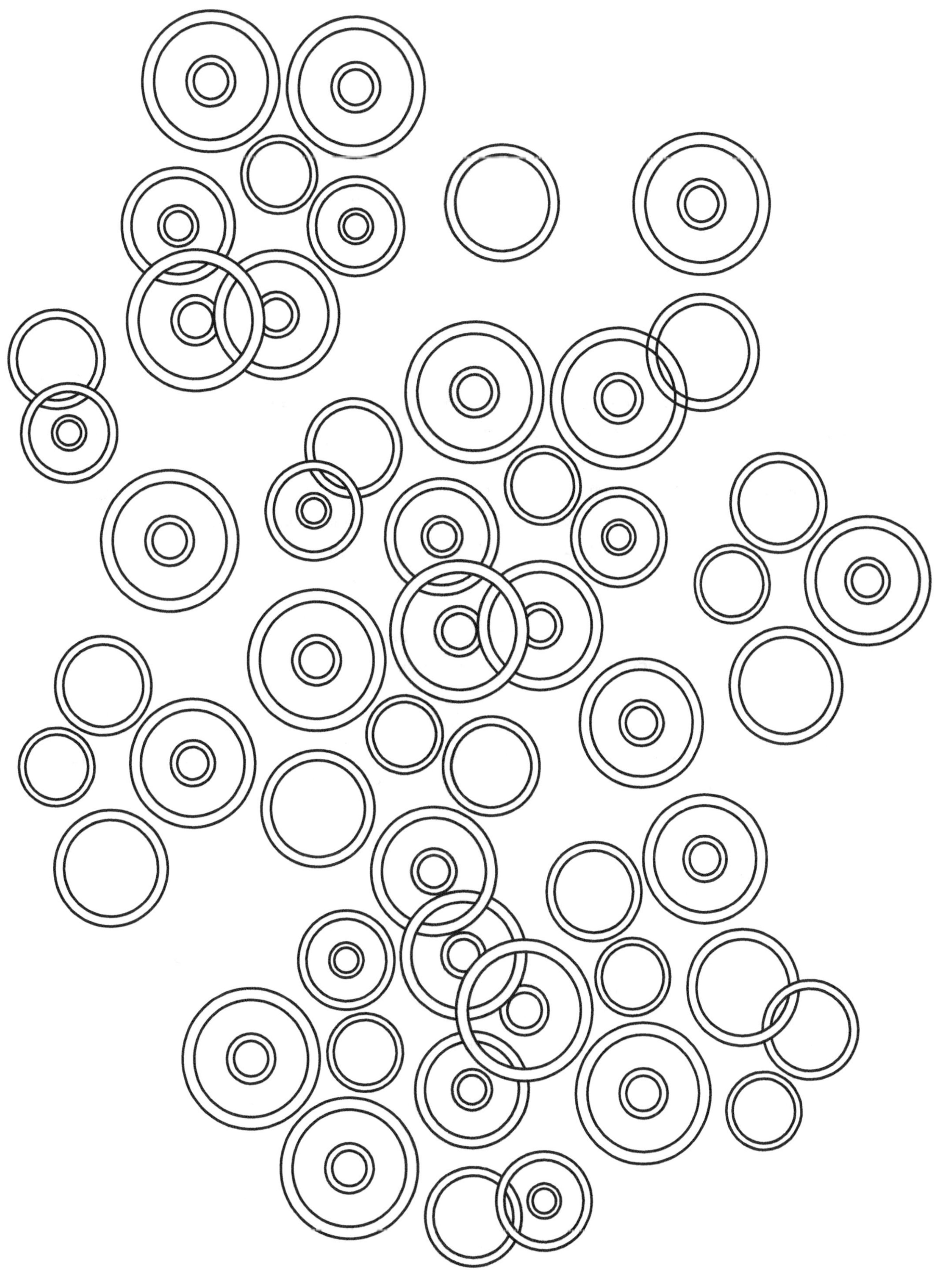

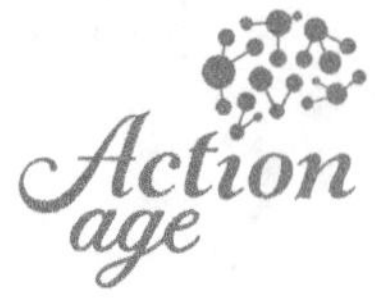

About Action Age

At Action Age, we aim to create, provide and track down resources for seniors, with a particular emphasis on those suffering from Dementia and Alzhiemer's.

By selling products, we are able to fund the creation of new products that make a meaningful impact for seniors, and continue the work done through our organization.

However, we understand that not every carer or family member has the financial capability to continually purchase products. Our primary objective is, and always will be, to improve and provide care to seniors. One way we achieve this (apart from physical care) is the creation of meaningful products.

If you have purchased this book, and found it useful but cannot afford another, or work at a dementia or Alzheimer's facility, please contact us and we can arrange discounted products for bulk sales for aged care facilities or printable versions to use at these facilities, and a sample of some of our other products. Please email or message us at the following locations, and mention that you purchased this book, and a bit abxout your situation!

hello@actionage.org
Facebook https://www.facebook.com/Actionage

Note: For those who receive any digital files from us, we maintain a strict copyright on the material. It is illegal to resell or reuse the file in part or as a whole, or forward the file digitally to anyone. You may only pass on or give out the file in PRINTED FORM.

How can you help us?

- **Please consider leaving an honest review on Amazon for any of our products that you purchase. This is one way of helping us grow!**
- Send us an email at hello@actionage.org and join our mailing list and receive free resources of Dementia and Alzhiemers care, as well as information about our new products or physical care updates
- Like our facebook page, again to receive free information, products and updates.

We really appreciate your purchase! Each purchase made helps fund our organisation and expand the number of people who receive our care!